EAT WELL

FOR $50 A WEEK

by Rhonda Barfield

Design by Michael Barfield
Photos by Ed Crim

Library of Congress Catalog Card Number: 93-090105

ISBN: 0-9635782-0-0

Although the author has carefully researched the information contained in this book, I cannot assume responsibility for errors, inaccuracies or omissions herein.

ACKNOWLEDGMENTS

My sincere thanks go to Nancy Castleman, Marc Eisenson, Marcy Ross, Jackie Iglehart, Candace Magruder and Anneliese Thomas for their thorough proofreading, constructive criticism and excellent suggestions. Many others — most of them named in the text — contributed by offering expert advice and information. I appreciate all the loving input.

Thank you, Mother, and mother-in-law Marilyn, for some wonderful recipes and cooking tips through the years. I am always inspired by your good examples of thriftiness.

I'm especially grateful to my husband and dearest friend, Michael, for his encouragement and many hours of babysitting. Thank you, too, Eric, Christian, Lisa and Mary, for putting up with Mom on the days when I tried to write, and you kept busy elsewhere!

Eat Well For $50 a Week is dedicated to those who need some extra cash — as we did — in order to accomplish the dreams in their lives.

FOREWORD

Shop with Rhonda and learn all her money saving tips in this book. It is bursting with expert advice for those who want to chop their food budgets in half. Both interesting and instructive, it contains sound, common sense ideas mixed with refreshing creativity. Whether you are a beginner in the kitchen or need to change old habits, choose from numerous budget trimming ideas, such as bulk buying from stores, belonging to a co-op, gleaning, gardening, couponing, refunding, bartering, using organizational techniques, and much more.

This book is a must for somebody like me. When my husband's income was slashed $25,000, cutting costs in the kitchen was a big part of our strategy that allowed us to still live within our means. Anyone hit by the recession can profit immensely from using the suggestions given here.

Like Rhonda, I also feed a family (five, including teenagers) on $50 a week, but I am going to post her checklist for savings in my kitchen to remind me to put her book into action, to motivate me to continue doing what works for us, and to help me remember that I am not alone in my endeavor to be frugal. If you are just starting to trim your budget, don't miss Chapter Four, where you will follow fictitious Penny Price for one year and learn how she trimmed her food budget week by week. Remember to take it one step at a time, then watch your savings grow!

Jackie Iglehart
Editor and Publisher, *The Penny Pincher Newsletter*

Contents

Introduction

Welcome to *Eat Well for $50 a Week*.

I'm not a professional writer, an outstanding cook, a nutritionist or a compulsive tightwad. My husband, four children and I live rather ordinary lives in a suburb of St. Louis. We're a typical Midwestern family.

As of this writing, Michael and I have been married for 19 years. We met in college, where I was a music education/speech major, and he was pursuing a degree in art. Like many others of our generation, upon graduation we discovered there really wasn't much one could do with a B.A. in fine arts.

For years we struggled along. We managed to stay debt-free, travel extensively and lead a contented lifestyle in spite of little money. And then we did something really foolish: we quit our jobs, gave notice on our apartment, put all our things in storage and left for a month-long back-packing trip. We had several good leads on future employment and were sure we could move right into solid careers after our vacationing was over.

It didn't work out that way at all. As we traveled around the country, our '69 Chevy broke down and had to be repaired. We charged those repairs, plus meals and some motel bills, on our credit cards. Our reasoning was that once we had jobs again, we could pay it all back quickly. The only trouble was, we were unemployed for nearly a year. During that time a friend in St. Louis offered us a place to stay while we got on our feet again. Unfortunately, by then we were heavily in debt.

Eventually I was hired to teach in a piano school and Michael free-lanced in art. Both of us were also employed by a temporary agency and picked up odd jobs wherever we could. One of my assignments led to a steady part-time position with an insurance company. We moved into a quiet, charming apartment complex. At last our lives were normalizing.

Then came children, four in six years, some planned, some not. Our medical bills mounted, and we were still paying on credit cards. I quit teaching, relying on the income and insurance benefits from my second job to pull us through. Michael went to work for a publishing company. When my part-time employer gave me an ultimatum — work full-time or be laid off — I chose to leave and stay home with the children.

In spite of serious money problems life was rather peaceful, at least for awhile. Then our apartment complex began to deteriorate, and rapidly. In one year's time the entire area changed, as newcomers moved in and most others moved out. Crime rose dramatically in our unstable neighborhood. There were rumors of a crack house down the street. Police patrols were everywhere, yet couldn't seem to control the problems. Burglary became commonplace. One night as we slept, someone nearly broke into our bedroom window.

We wanted to leave but simply didn't have the money. My parents generously lent us enough cash to cover a deposit and moving expenses, but how could we afford higher rent and utility bills on a regular basis? We analyzed our budget over and over again, trying to think of some way to squeeze out an extra hundred dollars or more a month.

At last we decided to cut back on groceries. It wasn't much, but we thought that by paring our spending from $80 to $100 down to $50 a week, we might be able to put aside just enough to afford better housing. At the same time we started our grocery budget, we also began an intensive search for a new home.

It took us seven months to find what we wanted: a large three-bedroom house with a bath and a half, huge fenced-in backyard, quiet neighborhood, dead-end street, and a large basement. We even have a garage, carport, laundry/mud room, central air, fireplace, attic fan and two garden spots. A delightful historic area is less than two miles away, and a hiking/biking trail a few blocks down the hill. The back yard is filled with trees and we have woods on two sides of our half-acre lot. This house could not have been more perfect for us! We now live in nearly four times the space we had before for $120 more a month. That's about what we're saving on groceries. As small as the dollar amount is, it has enabled us to have something much more important to us than steaks and microwave dinners.

My purpose in sharing my life story with you is to give some insight as to why I intentionally limit my weekly spending on food to $50, and why this self-imposed restraint is so important to me and my family. Many of you may be in a similar situation to ours. Perhaps you are living from paycheck to paycheck, laid off, unemployed or trying to survive on Social Security. *Eat Well For $50 a Week* will show you ways to cut back on nearly every item you buy, and the accumulated savings will enable you to eat well *and* have a little money left over.

On the other hand, many readers are looking for overall strategies that will help them save big. This is why I've included a crash course that explains bulk buying, couponing, refunding, co-ops, bartering, getting organized, making or cooking your own food, gardening, government programs and more. Chapters Two and Three tell you how to "beat the system," whether you do so at the store or elsewhere. The section on Resources provides valuable information, addresses and phone numbers to get you started.

Perhaps you've read all the theories behind saving on groceries, but can't understand how to really make it happen. You'll find help in Chapter Four, where a hypothetical family changes their lifestyle little by little, one change a week, for 52 weeks of the year. The results are big savings on their food budget.

You may think you have a good excuse — from following a low-cholesterol diet to catering to demanding children — for spending lots of money at the supermarket. If so, refer to Chapter Five. There may be an answer there for you.

Or take a look at Chapter One and Appendix Two, listings of my "real-life" shopping lists and menu plans for four weeks. I don't expect anyone to follow them to the letter, of course, but I hope they convince you that it is possible to eat well for $50 a week. We do! And there are six of us!

The U.S. Department of Agriculture says an American family of four (two adults, ages 20-50, and two children, one age six to eight, the other, nine to 11 years old) spends $82.80 for groceries weekly on a thrifty plan, $106.30 on a low-cost plan, $132.60 on a moderate-cost plan, and $159.70 on a liberal budget.* Their figures may be accurate for the

---

*From the Human Nutrition Information Service of USDA, December 1992. Updates are made monthly.

shopper who's strolling through a grocery store pulling items off the shelf. But if you're willing to work at your budget, you can cut even that low-cost bill in half.

Doesn't this all require an incredible amount of time and energy? Not as much as you might think. I can't answer the question categorically because I don't know how many hours you are now spending in shopping, meal planning and cooking. It takes me about an hour to devise a shopping list based on store specials, and about two hours to shop with my four chidren — Eric, 6; Christian, 5; Lisa, 3; and Mary, 18 months — in tow. I enjoy cooking, but between homeschooling my six year old, running a household and writing, I don't spend many hours in the kitchen. You'll find my recipes in Chapter Six to be mostly fast and easy dishes.

Nobody's perfect, and that includes me. Just like you, I have days when I'm sick of cooking and throw something fast (and maybe inferior) on the table. Just like yours, my children love sweets and at best tolerate vegetables, and I accommodate them to some degree. Occasionally we eat too much red meat and not enough whole grains. Sometimes we impulse-buy at the supermarket and don't think twice about the cost. If you're looking for a perfect example to follow, you will not find her here.

But I do think I have some wonderfully helpful advice to share. I know there are many, many people who can benefit from the information in this book. My hope is to show those who honestly need to save money a way to do just that.

What are the dreams in your life? Could a little extra cash help you achieve them? If so, the grocery budget is a good place to start. While it may not be possible to cut back immediately on house or car payments, you *can* economize on food, beginning today. If you are a typical family spending, say, $120 a week, scaling down to $50 is a $70 weekly savings, a $280 monthly savings, and a $3,640 yearly savings, all of it tax-free "income."

So with all this said, why not begin to *Eat Well for $50 a Week*?

Real-Life Shopping

When we began our $50 a week grocery budget, I found the hardest part was changing my old habits. I liked to ramble through the supermarket, toss a few items in the cart, and splurge on anything else that looked appealing. And I simply couldn't do that anymore. $50 plus impulse buying yielded two and a half bags of groceries! That was certainly not enough to feed a family of six for a week.

At the time I knew virtually nothing about bulk buying, couponing, refunding, co-ops, bartering, gardening, gleaning and other strategies mentioned in this and the next two chapters. I had to start with shopping at local stores and figure out a way to get the most for my money there.

During this transition period I heard about a publication by Donna McKenna, a teacher from Maine, who wrote *The $30 a Week Grocery Budget.* Donna was feeding two adults and four children for $20 less than I was. I ordered her booklet and read it cover to cover. It was an excellent starting point, and helped me devise my own system. Here's what I decided to do.

1. Set a limit on spending and stay under it with few exceptions.

2. Compare prices at nearby stores to see which store was least expensive overall.

3. Buy most of our groceries from the cheapest store.

4. Supplement by shopping at other stores whose weekly specials were outstanding.

5. Make a detailed shopping list and follow it to the letter, substituting only when unexpected bargains justified a change.

Does this sound complicated? It isn't. Let me explain each point in more detail.

1. Set a limit on spending.

It's been my experience that if I allow myself $75, I spend that much just as easily as I spend $50. Restricting my outlay helped me to think creatively about possibilities. I had to examine my priorities carefully. Did I really need to buy juice boxes for the children, or expensive breakfast cereals? Was there a cheaper substitute? What helped most was thinking of the budget as an adventure rather than a toilsome burden. How *much* could I buy for $50? — that was my objective. It became a kind of game to try and get more for my money each week.

Nobody says you have to spend what I spend. You may actually have to go lower, or you may find $100 a much more comfortable range. Limiting yourself is still important. It makes you feel in control of your budget and forces you to use money wisely.

2. Compare prices.

I memorized about a hundred prices, not because I planned to, but just because I was interested. You don't need to, of course; it's easier and more helpful to keep a "price book" with the cost of items you buy regularly. For example, your notebook might look something like this:

Store	5 lbs. sugar	5 lbs. flour	1 lb. stick margarine
Natl.	Name Brand, 2.29	Name Brand, 1.19	Name Brand, .99
	Store Brand, 1.99	Store Brand, .89	Store Brand, .89
	Generic, 1.79	Generic, .79	Generic, none
A&P	Name Brand, 2.19	Name Brand, 1.19	Name Brand, .89
	Store Brand, 2.09	Store Brand, .99	Store Brand, none
	Generic, none	Generic, .89	Generic, none

On the line above across from National, I have recorded brand name prices, line two is store brand, and line three is generic. To compile the information, you can do all your shopping at National one week and quickly jot down prices as you buy. Next week do the same at A&P, and so on until you've completed a price list for several stores. The store with the overall lowest costs will be your new base store.

Supermarkets are only one possibility. I checked out discount and wholesale grocers, food co-ops, day-old bakeries, produce stands, farmers' markets, dairies, buying clubs, cheese factory outlets, meat markets and health food stores. There was a wealth of information in our big-city yellow pages under Grocers and Food. Even if you live in a more rural area, I think

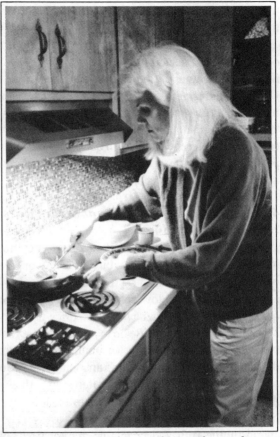

Homemade oatmeal pancakes make a cheap, nutritious breakfast.

you'll be surprised at what you may find in your phone book. Also talk to friends and neighbors about good buys in your area, wherever you live. I've gotten some great leads just by asking around.

3. Buy most groceries from the cheapest store.

This may seem so obvious it's hardly worth mentioning. It's surprising, though, how many people prefer to shop someplace that offers them spotlessly waxed floors and every imaginable convenience. I understand. But such stores are usually not the places where you'll save the most money.

My personal favorite is Aldi, a no-frills discount warehouse that offers a limited selection, but at 50% to 80% below most supermarket prices.* It's amazing how much cheaper some stores are than others. Many products at Aldi, for example, cost less than supermarket brand names advertising a half-price savings! In other words, when National's "special" on potato chips is 89 cents, Aldi's store brand price is 59 cents (with little difference, if any, in quality). This is why it is so important to price check by referring to your notebook, then select a store that can supply most of your needs economically.

4. Supplement by shopping at other stores whose weekly specials are outstanding.

Did you know that supermarkets sometimes take a loss on a few items in order to entice you to buy there? "Loss leader" specials — some or all of those advertised on the front and back of weekly fliers — may actually be priced below cost. You can easily spot the real bargains by quickly leafing through several ads, price notebook in hand. It takes me about ten minutes to decide on my second store for the week, based on the items I need that are on sale. In another ten minutes I've combed through that store's ad a second time and am ready to write down my shopping list.

I won't say it's easy, but I often stop at three or more stores a week. All three are generally within a five mile radius of my home, and bargains have to be incredible to lure me farther away. The children and I usually swing by the fruit and vegetable market first. Next we shop at either Schnucks or National, then Aldi. Sometimes we also walk right next door to the butcher's or a penny candy store. Even with a six year old, two preschoolers and a toddler trailing along (and helping me), our entire excursion takes about two hours.

---

*Aldi is located only in Midwestern states as of this writing, but the company plans to expand into Pennsylvania, New Jersey, New York, Maryland, Tennessee and Kentucky in 1993 and 1994. See Resources for a complete listing of current divisional headquarters' numbers. (They are not found in many phone books.) I have also just discovered Save-A-Lot Food Stores, comparable to Aldi and available in some states where Aldi is not. See Resources.

5. Make a detailed shopping list.

As I write down items I need for the week, I try to match up ideas for meals with store specials. If pork is on sale, for example, I will plan to buy and serve that instead of higher-priced meat. Our menus are flexible so that I can take advantage of cheaper foods.

My shopping list starts with essentials, and then I add other foods I would also like to buy. I estimate the total cost for everything on my list, then subtract coupon values. If I'm under $50 I can add more; if over, I have to delete a few things. Sometimes I take a little extra money with me just in case. But most days I'm within a dollar or two of my estimate.

Substitutions are justified when I find an unexpected good deal. One day last year, Aldi had marked down all their 2% milk to $1.00 a gallon. I crossed some long-term baking items off my list and bought a few extra jugs, some set aside until the following week.

But in order to demonstate just how my system works, I want to share an actual shopping list and menu plans for the week of July 15th through the 21st, 1992.* First I'll detail the list and the total prices, then I'll explain why I bought what I did. (Items are arranged in approximate categories as I knew I needed them.) Menu plans follow.

SHOPPING LIST

From Aldi

3 gallons 2% milk	2 8-ounce packages mozzarella cheese
10-ounce package colby cheese	2 pounds stick margarine
1 large container sour cream	1 small container strawberry yogurt
2 dozen eggs	1 large bag corn chips
1 large bag tortilla chips	1 large bag potato chips
1 large bag pretzels	1 box graham crackers
1 box macaroni and cheese dinner	1 can chicken noodle soup
1 can cream of chicken soup	2 packages dry onion soup
2 pounds brown sugar	1 can water-packed tuna
1 large jar Prego spaghetti sauce	1 can cooking spray
1 large jar applesauce	1 container whipped topping

*Actually, I've kept track of *four* consecutive weeks of shopping lists and menu plans. For those of you who'd like to read more, see Appendix Two for three more weeks' worth of shopping lists and menus.

1 can frozen orange juice conc.	2 packages deli turkey
1 can biscuits	1 package English muffins
2 loaves whole wheat bread	1 box store brand toasted oats cereal
1 box puffed wheat cereal	1 head lettuce
Total: $30.48	

From Shop 'n Save

1 whole watermelon	1 tomato
4 large apples	4 large oranges
4 pounds bananas	3 potatoes
2 large bunches grapes	6 ears sweet corn
1 can baking powder	1 package flour tortillas
Total: $8.13	

From C. Rallo Meat Company

1 pound slab bacon	3 pounds chuck roast
Total: $5.20	

Grand Total: $43.81*

As you can see from my list, I buy a lot of what you probably buy. Aldi sells mostly private label goods. With prices on chips and crackers about one-third or less of regular supermarket prices, I purchase three to four bags a week as a lunch supplement. I occasionally splurge on Prego brand spaghetti sauce (still much cheaper at Aldi) because I have never been able to duplicate the delicious taste through home cooking or doctoring other brands.

You may wonder why I purchase only one carton of yogurt and one can of soup. Sometimes I split the yogurt between the four children (the baby eats a teaspoonful), adding diced bananas. I may stretch the soup with leftover meats and vegetables, just enough to provide a light meal.

The second store mentioned is a little more out of my way than others and I usually don't shop there. But this particular week, the produce department was engaged in a price war with another store. I was able to

---

*I have saved all my receipts for these weeks and will gladly supply a photocopy to skeptics.

buy two bags of groceries at about 50% less than usual.

The meat market is rather expensive but right next door to Aldi. I make it a point to buy whatever is on sale, if anything. This week the specials were not outstanding, so I relied more heavily on what was in my home freezer. Several days before, I stocked up on chicken leg quarters at 29 cents a pound, cooked a big batch in the Crock-Pot, boned them and froze the pieces. I also had turkey and fish sticks on hand.

Perhaps you noticed that my shopping list does not include any non-food items, like disposable diapers, aluminum foil, paper towels and laundry detergent. I generally buy them at Aldi. The $4.99-a-bag diapers, for example, are a weekly expenditure. The rest I usually purchase twice a month. We try to make do with reusable goods, such as cloth rather than paper napkins, whenever possible. I even recycle some very carefully-washed foil. I have not recorded anything other than food, but even with these items figured in, my average weekly grocery bill is still $50.00 to $55.00 or less.

Here are the menus for breakfast, lunch, dinner and two daily snacks — real-life menus, remember! — that followed from my shopping.

WEEKLY MENU

July 15

    B: Cold cereal with milk
    S: Graham crackers
    L: Nachos with melted cheese and salsa, bananas and grapes, milk
    S: Orange juice
    D: Chuck roast*, carrots, potatoes and gravy, chocolate cookies

July 16

    B: Oatmeal and granola*, raisins, milk
    S: Bananas and grapes
    L: Peanut butter and jelly sandwiches on whole wheat bread, corn chips, milk
    S: Watermelon slices
    D: Stir-fry with chicken and garden vegetables*, rice, poppy seed muffins*

July 17

B: Scrambled eggs, toast, milk
S: Orange juice popsicles
L: Macaroni and cheese, pretzels, canned pears, milk
S: Caramel corn*
D: Hot dogs and hamburgers, carrot sticks, grapes, caramel corn*

July 18

B: Oatmeal pancakes*
S: Bananas
L: Chicken noodle soup, crackers, raisins, milk
S: Watermelon slices
D: Turkey, dry bread dressing*, gravy*, corn on the cob, wacky cake*

July 19

B: Cold cereal with milk
S: Sliced apples
L: Leftovers, milk
S: Orange juice popsicles
D: Dinner out at Taco Bell

July 20

B: Oatmeal and granola*, milk
S: Grapes and bananas
L: Biscuit pizzas, animal crackers, milk
S: Watermelon slices
D: Bacon sandwiches with homemade French bread*, lettuce wedges, tomatoes, zucchini, sweet French salad dressing*, sugar cookies

July 21

B: Toast and scrambled eggs, milk
S: Bananas
L: Leftovers, milk
S: Orange juice popsicles
D: Fish sticks, popovers*, corn, marshmallow treats

*Starred items can be found in Recipes. To locate an exact page number, refer to the Recipe Index on page 144.

Let me explain the preceding menus in a little more detail. Our food is pretty basic. We eat few casseroles and soups because Eric, Christian and Lisa simply don't like them. Although we serve meat nearly every day at dinner, our per-serving size is generally only a few ounces. Instead we offer large portions of breads, pastas, rice and vegetables. Our meals are not only low-cost but also, for the most part, nutritious.

I make it a point to see that my children have at least three one-cup servings of milk or milk products, one generous serving of vitamin C and two servings each of fruits and vegetables daily. This may not be obvious when reading through the menus. For example, on "cereal days" the children usually eat two or three bowls of cold cereal, getting at least two milk servings each at those breakfasts. Sometimes, instead of orange juice, we spread out the vitamin C in grapes, watermelon, tomatoes, etc. throughout the day. At dinner we generally have double portions of one favorite vegetable, or I may add diced or pureed zucchini, onion or peppers to a meat dish and disguise both the taste and appearance. Stir-fry with chicken and garden vegetables, served on July 16th, offered just such an opportunity.

We enjoy dessert nearly every night, as all of us have a sweet tooth. I am certain we could save money if we skipped the sugary finale to our

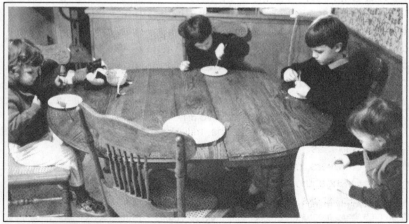

The Barfield children finish up a healthy breakfast — pancakes — at a cost of about 15¢ per person (store-bought cereal can run as high as $1.00 per person).

meals, but it's not something we're willing to give up just yet. Instead, we are trying to convert to more healthful desserts.

I am not trying to justify my menus nor insist that you follow them. Hopefully these listings will give you an idea of exactly what I do and do not serve within the restraints of my $50 budget. Please don't think I'm suggesting that you eat just as we do. If you are interested in more "health food" or vegetarian meals, refer to *More-with-Less Cookbook,* listed in Resources.

You will recall I promised *real-life* menus. It was very tempting to doctor these listings and show you perfectly balanced meals. Unfortunately, I don't always succeed in feeding us ideally. At one point, I considered recording menus as I *planned* to serve them, a model for the month, so to speak. But I thought it might be more helpful to play "true confessions" and tell you what we really ate for four weeks.* I trust you will not imitate my deficiencies!

On July 17th the restaurant next door to us advertised 25 cent hot dogs and hamburgers, and we just couldn't pass up the low prices. We eat out once or twice every two weeks, as restaurant dining with the family is an important part of our entertainment. If you think I'm being unfair not including this in the food budget, then I'll accommodate you and add in the extra $13 we spent on tacos; that still puts our weekly food budget at $56.81!

They say it takes 21 days to break a habit. I think it took a little longer for me to get used to a new way of shopping and spending less, then planning and cooking lower-cost meals. But now — as I type on our new computer system, listen to the children playing downstairs in our large basement and watch the fire crackling in the hearth — it certainly seems worth the effort. "Depriving" ourselves of a few groceries has enabled us to have many other things that we've enjoyed much more.

---

*I submitted my menu plans to a registered dietician for analysis. Here is her comment: "Although these menus may not exactly meet all of the recommended dietary guidelines, when balancing budget, food preferences of children and dietary considerations, they are adequate and realistic." Melanie Gillingham, MS, RD

2

Beat The System At The Store

*T*wo years ago I really didn't know much about saving money on food. Since then, I've discovered ways to "beat the supermarket system" through careful buying of loss leader sale items, marked-down meat and produce, and day-old bread. I've also learned more about bulk buying at warehouse stores, large-scale couponing and refunding. Today, I get a lot more for my money than I used to!

As I mentioned in the last chapter, there are all sorts of retail and wholesale outlets — grocery stores, markets, buying clubs, warehouses and more — where you can purchase low-cost groceries. The trick is to beat the system at that particular store.

SAVE MONEY ON WHAT YOU BUY

Let's assume that you've already chosen a base store and are ready to do some serious shopping. Here are some guidelines for saving money on specific foods.

Meats

Watch carefully for sales and stock up on the feature of the week. Buy a month's worth of chicken at 39 cents a pound, and next week a month's worth of beef roast for half price.

When turkeys and hams go on sale during Thanksgiving and Christmas, try to have enough money set aside to invest in more than one for your freezer.

Consider buying meat in quantity. You may be able to purchase half a side of beef at the meat market for a price 50% less than the supermarket's. Find a few friends with freezer space, and you're all set.

Buy fish or seafood that is currently in season.

Rely on cheaper turkey or chicken cold cuts and hot dogs rather than those made from beef and pork.

Ask meat managers if they offer discounts on the ends of deli meats or mark down older cuts. I have located one local store that sells surplus meat at half price, and less.

Cost compare, and you may be able to buy on-sale meat from a butcher. If so, ask him to give you the bones and other throw-aways along with the prime cuts; you can make them into soups and broths.

Dairy Foods

Purchasing milk products at the supermarket can be expensive, but there are other options. You may have to shop around to find the best prices. Start with a food warehouse or buyer's club, Aldi, or Save-A-Lot. Can you locate a dairy or cheese outlet store through your local yellow pages? Even driving some distance for milk products may be worth a once-a-month trip, especially if you buy in large quantities and freeze milk and cheese.

Many dairy foods — milk substitutes, soft margarine, low-fat sour cream and yogurt — can be made cheaply from scratch. See the Recipe Index for ideas.

Produce

As a rule, don't buy fresh fruits and vegetables at the supermarket unless you can find them as "loss leaders." Keep your eyes open and you should be able to locate a produce stand in your area, one that stays open year round. I used to frequent a stand where "loose" grapes and slightly bruised apples were sold at 75% off the regular low prices. Sometimes such bargains are not readily apparent, so you should be inquisitive.

Wherever you shop, purchase only what's in season and/or on sale. Apples, of course, are common in the fall, as are pumpkins and winter squash. Oranges and grapefruits peak in November through April. Strawberries are best in late spring. See the chart on page 112 for detailed information.

Wherever you shop, ask the produce manager if he or she would be willing to set out bags of "browner" bananas at half price. Find out what he or she does with damaged produce and volunteer to buy it cheap (or better yet, haul it off for free).

Weigh bagged produce to find the one that's slightly heavier. You may discover a two pound bag, for example, that holds two and a half pounds of carrots.

Try to process older and damaged produce immediately for maximum nutrition and minimum waste. If leafy vegetables are wilted, pick off the brown edges, sprinkle with cool water, wrap in a towel and refrigerate. You can freeze most fruits and vegetables in airtight containers or freezer bags; consult a standard cookbook for more specific advice.

Fresh produce is best for you. Canned fruits and vegetables have less nutritional value and a higher sodium content than frozen or fresh equivalents. But if you must rely on canned produce, look for store brand, generic, or on-sale name brands whenever possible. Those who cook in large quantities should consider buying institutional size cans of vegetables, which are often much cheaper per ounce than their smaller counterparts. Another alternative is to purchase generic frozen vegetables, then steam them in a covered saucepan; the cost will probably be higher, but so will the vitamin content.

Breads, Grains, Pasta, Cereals

I used to buy all my bread from a day-old bakery, saving about 50% over supermarket prices. Now I purchase fresh whole wheat loaves at Aldi for even less than that. Compare prices carefully in your area to find the best, low-cost source.

If you do purchase day-old breads, try to stock up on varieties that can be easily reheated. Slightly tough rolls, for example, taste delicious when oven-browned until crispy. Or try my mother-in-law's trick: she heats water in a large pan on the stove, adds a wire basket filled with day-old bread, and steams the bread briefly until hot and tender.

Many whole grain products are actually quite cheap, such as oats, Cream of Wheat cereal and corn meal. Bulk buy these and your baking supplies — flour, yeast, spices, etc. — as well as beans, rice and pasta, if possible. You may want to freeze grains overnight, then seal in airtight containers. If 50 pound quantities far exceed your needs, again, consider sharing with friends.

BULK BUY FROM WAREHOUSE STORES

Recently Michael and I were given a free membership in a wholesale club just down the road. Sam's Club has good prices and good quality. So we tried stocking up on, among other things, Captain Crunch cereal and tortilla chips.

It was fun while it lasted. The only trouble was, it didn't last as long as it was supposed to. For us, buying ten times our normal amount of chips did *not* mean we had chips ten times as long. It meant we ate a lot more a lot faster. Our problem with buying in bulk is that we tend to eat in bulk, too.

It is not this way for everyone. I know of some families who visit the wholesale club, stock-up stores and other outlets once a month, buy wisely, and then consume wisely. Stocking up on items like yeast, for example, makes sense: you can keep it tucked away in the refrigerator, and can't sit down in front of the TV and overindulge in it. Jackie Iglehart (publisher of *The Penny Pincher*) purchases bulk flour from a bakery owner, and so is able to make homemade bread for pennies a loaf. Smart bulk buying like this amounts to huge savings.

Adrianne Ferree (former publisher of *The Frugal Times*) offers good advice in her second issue, "Grocery Warehouse Do's and Don'ts." Here are some of her suggestions:

➤ Don't buy products just to try out at home. Make sure you really like and will use the product.

➤ Don't buy products you can get cheaper elsewhere.

➤ Don't buy products that supposedly save you money if you're spending more in the long run by buying more (e.g., my tortilla chips story).

➤ Don't buy margarine, canned vegetables, meats, standard sodas and bread at the warehouse, as you can usually find them at cost or below at supermarkets, especially with use of double coupons.

➤ Do look around on your first visit. Note prices, unit costs and quantities before you buy.

➤ Do go at a time that's less hectic than rush hour.

➤ Do make a list and stick to it. Don't allow yourself to linger and be tempted.

➤ Do buy just enough to last until your next visit. In the meantime, you will probably be able to use other shopping strategies that might save you more money.

One more word on bulk buying from stores: try to keep extra money set aside for the best bargains. Check stores regularly for damaged goods and loss leader items. Buy as much as you can possibly afford when the price is right.

For a listing of warehouse membership clubs nationwide, see Appendix One.

USE COUPONS

Maybe you're looking for additional ways to save money at the supermarket. If so, large-scale couponing and/or refunding may be the answer for you.

Cheapskate Monthly newsletter featured a woman who claims to have "saved solely with coupons and refunds a total of...*$17,433.17*" since 1980! Twice a week, Mary Ann Maring spends at least an hour scanning the ads for local supermarkets, clipping store coupons and determining the best buys for what she needs. Next she goes through her extensive files, matching up manufacturers' coupons with sales and store coupons wherever possible. To keep current, Mary Ann purges her files every four months. Expired coupons are pitched, and soon-to-expire ones are rotated to the front of each category.

$17,000 is a lot of money. I found Mary Ann's approach intriguing: she has learned to play the couponing game to great personal advantage. As *Cheapskate Monthly* notes, "There were many items for which she would pay only a few cents and occasionally she pointed out an item she would be getting absolutely *free!*"

Once in awhile I do use coupons. Recently at the supermarket I

25

picked up two candy bars for five cents each, five cans of name brand vegetables for 60 cents total, and two bottles of Softsoap for 60 cents each. I know couponing works. But I must admit I don't think, generally speaking, it merits a significant investment of my time.

For example, by using coupons the Del Monte vegetables cost 15 cents a can. The same size private label corn is 19 cents a can at my base store, Aldi. I honestly can't tell a difference in taste. And to save four cents a can, I had to find a store featuring Del Monte vegetables on sale, clip a coupon, search the shelves a few moments to find an exact match, and redeem a double coupon. Maybe I dislike all of this bother because of four children hurrying me along. I want things quick and easy, and the extra work for four pennies is simply not worth it to me.

And here's another problem. Most coupons are printed for highly packaged convenience foods, like expensive, ready-to-eat cereal or salad dressings. So even if I buy on sale with double coupons, I may still pay more for an item that I can make myself.

At the grocery store this week I did a cost comparison of three items at original price and after double coupons, contrasting with both a name brand and Aldi's brand. (I assume you could find similar prices at a warehouse store in your area.) Here's what I discovered:

Lucky Charms cereal costs $3.69; with a 50 cent coupon doubled, $2.69. But I can buy a similar product, same size, at Aldi for $1.69. Or I can serve my family oatmeal for breakfast for less than 50 cents!

Yoplait yogurt costs 69 cents; with a "30 cents off 2" coupon doubled, 39 cents each; at Aldi, yogurt is 29 cents for the same size; and homemade may be even cheaper.

Log Cabin Syrup costs $3.29; with a 40 cent coupon doubled, $2.49; Aldi's version is 79 cents for a smaller size, or $1.58 for two equaling the Log Cabin bottle; and homemade costs 80 cents or less.

If saving money is your main goal, you would have to locate these items on sale and double a coupon to even approach the cost of the homemade products.

Still, couponing may be a viable option for you if you think of it as a hobby, enjoy name brand products, or have a difficult time finding discounted food. Here are some tips from Charlotte Gorman, author of *The Frugal Mind,* Jackie Iglehart of *The Penny Pincher* newsletter, and

Mary Kenyon, an expert couponer:

- Subscribe to the Sunday newspaper, a great source of coupons. Also check the food section of the daily paper, women's magazines, and boxes at the front of some supermarkets.

- Ask willing friends and relatives to save coupons for you. Consider setting up a coupon exchange box at the library.

- Look over couponing magazines (see Resources under "Refunding") to decide whether a subscription is worth your while.

- Clip all coupons and file them in appropriate categories, such as Breads, Cleaning Products, Frozen Foods, etc..

- Make a coupon file from a small box, tabbed and divided by cardboard pieces. Always take your coupon box along when you leave home.

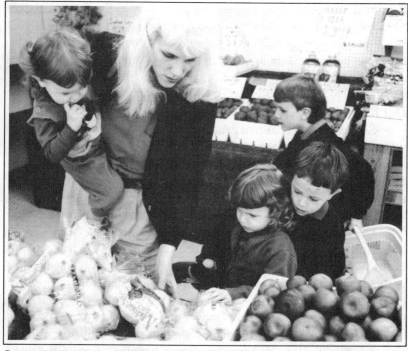

Sunnyside Produce offers quality fruits and vegetables at a 50% savings over regular supermarket prices. Check your area for similar stands and stores.

- Decide ahead of time what coupons you will use at the store, and transfer them to an envelope. Arrange the coupons in the order that you find foods placed in store aisles, on your usual route, by supermarket aisles, or alphabetically.

- Don't buy items just because you have a coupon unless it's something you'd use anyway, or unless it's free or nearly free.

- Besides buying on sale, try to use coupons for products that you find in damaged or discontinued bins.

- Stockpile when you find a particularly good deal.

Cheapskate Monthly suggests you may be an excellent candidate for couponing if you like to organize things, have tenacity and patience, can see the big picture, are flexible and enjoy a challenge.

But if you're thinking, as I am, that this is just too much work, then large-scale couponing may not be for you. Says Amy Dacyzyn, author of *The Tightwad Gazette*, "I feel that using couponing and refunding as your major grocery strategy will reduce your food bill, but not as much as if you use a combination of strategies." In the end, it comes down to personal preference.

DO REFUNDING

Some of us have taken advantage of a refund offer or two. Perhaps we've dutifully clipped the UPC symbol from a box of cereal, mailed it in, and received a check for $1.00 in the mail. I never found myself too enthusiastic about a return of a couple of bucks a month, especially considering the work and postage involved. Then again, there *are* ways to use refunding as a major means of saving money on groceries.

The Tightwad Gazette describes a remarkable woman, Mary Kenyon of Independence, Iowa, who spends about $385 monthly to feed a family of six. What's remarkable about it? Well, Mary saves an average of 20% of that amount through coupon use, and receives back *$110* each month on refunds, even after postage! That brings her weekly grocery bill down to $50.

I gave Mary a call to learn more. She tells me that she is now saving almost 30% off the cost of food through couponing. But what I really wanted to know about was refunding: exactly how does one get back all that money? Mary wrote:

"I save all my labels, receipts and UPC symbols and file them in Ziploc bags according to product categories (i.e., juice, aspirin, cereal, crackers). I have two file cabinets and shelves with boxes to hold my qualifiers. I have several traders (other refunders) who I regularly trade refund forms and complete deals with. This way I am able to take advantage of many more refunds that are put out by manufacturers each month.... I spend 15-20 hours a week working on refunding, in 15 minute to half-hour stretches. This includes clipping and sorting coupons, planning a grocery list, cutting and filing qualifiers, sending out for refunds and organizing trades."

What does all this effort get Mary? "I provide 85% of my children's Christmas gifts through my refunding," Mary explained. "I usually have extra t-shirts and watches to give to my brothers and have also given baskets of trial-size products and food products I've gotten free with coupons to my mother, a sister or an elderly shut-in." In addition, "After postage ($15.00 to $20.00 a month), I average $90.00 in cash, another $25.00 to $35.00 in free product coupons, and five to 20 free gifts back. If you subtract that $90.00 in cash from what I spent on groceries, then I really did save a great deal."

Michele Easter, publisher of *Refunding Makes Cents! (RMC)*, says, "I receive many checks in the mail *every month* by taking the time to peel labels, cut off UPCs, and mail away for cash, gifts and free coupons. I mail for at least 100 refunds every month on all types of household products. So my mailbox is stuffed with checks for $1, $5, $10, and more, and I receive free t-shirts, toys, tapes, etc., plus wonderful coupons for free full size products."

I scanned the pages of the November 1992 *RMC*, and was impressed with both the scope and complexity of the bulletin. But I must confess I still have my doubts about refunding. For example, here is a typical offer from page 12:

"10 free jars of Gerber 1st, 2nd or 3rd Foods Baby Foods. Send 48 UPCs from Gerber baby foods or juices." 48 jars of baby food, at an average price of 50 cents each, adds up to $24.00. You get ten free jars and so supposedly save $5.00. It all sounds impressive until you consider that 48 meals of a homemade equivalent, whipped up in the blender from your own delicious food, would only cost a few dollars or less. Which makes more sense, to not spend much money in the first place, or to spend a fair amount, then work at least an hour to get some back? Refunders claim big savings, but for my family, most of the time, it doesn't make cents *or* sense.

Here's another offer listed in *RMC*:

"Free mermaid doll. Send five UPCs from Chicken of the Sea products for a free doll...." Oh yes, and there *is* a $1.95 postage and handling fee. So I buy five cans of name brand tuna at 89 cents each (the cheapest Chicken of the Sea product I could find), add p&h and arrive at a figure of $6.40 needed for my "free" doll. Wouldn't it be simpler, and much cheaper, to buy generic tuna at 49 cents a can? And pick up a mermaid doll — as we did — at a garage sale for a quarter? My total cost for five cans of tuna *and* a doll is $2.70. Who's really saving money here, not to mention time?

Refunders will argue that it's not that simple, that UPCs can be traded for free or rescued from the trash, and food can be bought on sale in conjunction with coupons. The system is rather complicated and I haven't quite figured it out. Yet I have to give coupon queens like Michele Easter some benefit of the doubt: she and her 17,000 subscribers obviously make it work for themselves.

Charlotte Gorman, author of *The Frugal Mind*, is another expert who refunds. She prefers a detailed system of organizing offers and qualifiers. Charlotte writes down information about everything she sends for and notes the date. If nothing shows up in the mailbox within 12 weeks, she makes it a point to call or write the company's corporate headquarters.

Refund forms can be found in the same places as coupons, and also on bulletin boards in stores, at courtesy desks, on specially marked packages, and even at cashiers' counters. To learn more about refunding, refer to the publications listed in Resources.

So there you have it, several ways to beat the system at the store. And did you know there are other strategies you can use to cut your grocery bill, even without setting foot in a supermarket? Chapter Three shows you how.

3

Other Ways To Beat The System

*O*ne of the frustrating aspects of writing this book is that just when I think I've covered it all, new information comes in. Consider these ways to save on food: belonging to a co-op, bartering, organizing better for better savings, making or cooking more of your own food, gardening, gleaning, using government programs, and eating sensibly. If you don't enjoy shopping at grocery stores — or can't save as much as you'd like to there — then several other cost-cutting options are available to you.

BELONG TO A COOPERATIVE

I used to think of co-ops as groups of outdated hippie-type people who dined on unpalatable organic food. Ridiculous, I know, but I confess this stereotype lingered in the back of my mind.

When I began to seriously investigate cooperatives, it was a pleasant surprise to meet ordinary folks who were enthusiastic about their work. The National Cooperative Business Association, for example, offers a listing of helpful publications you can buy to learn more about co-ops. I called NCBA and requested their free how-to-get-started packet, finding it very informative. One article listed several advantages of a food buying co-op. Here are a few:

1. To support and invest in a business committed to local and organic food production and democratic control.

2. To eliminate much of the packaging involved in supermarket foods.

3. To meet and socialize with neighbors.

Other advantages can be savings on organic foods, at least over health food store prices. I consulted a catalog from Blooming Prairie Warehouse in Iowa City, Iowa, supplier for nearly a dozen co-ops in the St. Louis area. Selection is large and varied. Local co-op contact person Laurie Lowe explained, "Many members are concerned not only with cost, but also in buying quality organic and natural products." Laurie particularly likes the delicious cheese she purchases through Blooming Prairie.

Just how does a co-op operate? Jane Dewey, Sales Manager at Northeast Cooperative, says they're "community groups that pool their resources to buy groceries and produce in wholesale quantities at wholesale prices. Participating in a pre-order co-op involves ordering food in advance of the delivery, consolidating household orders into a group order, placing the order with a wholesaler, unloading it from the delivery truck, breaking it down into household orders, collecting payment and keeping accounting records."*

Most wholesalers do require a minimum order of at least $500, but several families buying together can add up dollars quickly. The more you order, the more you save.

It sounds a little involved to me. But Blooming Prairie assures its members that they will receive plenty of help, including access to technical and computer support, a lending library, meetings and seminars, a newsletter and more. The 150 page, fine-print catalog goes into great detail: it tells you if any given food is fruit juice-sweetened, has salt, wheat or yeast in it, and meets organics standards.

Joining a food buying co-op requires involvement. Depending on the organization, you may be asked to help recruit members, plan meetings, order, do paper work, bag, divide into individual orders and more. Some storefront co-ops request their members wait on customers in the store. And others will allow you to forego all the work if you're willing to pay more.

Finding the time to help may be a problem. Because many families these days have very few spare hours, the Michigan Federation had at one time "introduced a new type of buying club, in which a coordinator is paid 9% of the sales of the club for doing all of the work," says Joel David Welty, author of several publications on co-ops. "For some clubs, this can

*Reprinted from *NCBA Cooperative Business Journal*

mean extra income of $450 a month for the coordinator."* You organize and run the co-op, you get the price breaks *and* a commission. This may be an option for some.

As with any kind of food buying, self-restraint is a must. Take convenience foods, for example: co-ops offer them, just as the supermarket does. In Blooming Prairie's November/December 1992 catalog I found items as diverse as "Raviolini with Vermont Cheddar and Walnuts", "Jumbo Oat Bran Fruit Bars" and "Jammin' Corn and Potato Chowder." Whatever its form, recipe or brand name, a convenience food is still more expensive than making it yourself. Those who purchase through a co-op must be just as shrewd in their purchases as those who buy at stores.

Does belonging to a co-op really save you money? That depends, according to personal preferences. Is it important to you to purchase organic raisins? Are you allergic to milk, and presently buying soy substitutes at a health food store? Do you use canola oil — rather than generic vegetable oil — in your cooking? Then a co-op may be a cost-saving option.

On the other hand, if your eating habits are more "mainstream American," you'll need to take a close look at what co-ops sell and how that relates to what you buy. Also remember that some, though not all, local organizations charge membership fees. Once informed, you'll be able to make an intelligent decision about whether or not cooperatives might save you money on your weekly grocery bill.

I have to admit that researching co-ops has made me reconsider joining one myself. Blooming Prairie's catalog contains especially good prices on some items I regularly use, like yeast and spices. They also offer "deep discount deals" each month. Buying in case stack volume may yield discounts ranging from 10 to 30 percent. You can even order a sample package of several foods (usually new industry products) to try for a low price. And then there's that good cheese I keep hearing about....

If you're interested, refer to Resources (U.S. Cooperative Food Warehouses) to locate a co-op in your area. Maybe I'll see you at the next meeting.

*Reprinted from *NCBA Cooperative Business Journal*

BARTER

Years ago, when I taught piano lessons, I bartered a semester's worth of lessons for several pounds of prime Wisconsin cheese. My student's father owned a cheese factory, so it was a real bargain for her and a lot of delicious free food for me.

One-on-one bartering is not uncommon. But now there's a new, more complicated twist: trade networks that help businesses to work with each other on a non-cash basis. *USA Today* says: "Several firms dominate the barter market — each with its own rules. Generally, companies join a trade exchange, which offers their products or services at full price to other members of the exchange. They receive trade dollars in exchange, which they can spend on items they need."*

N.C.E.

Our neighbors, specialists in chimney repair, told me about National Commercial Exchange. The Bufords had just joined N.C.E. Already they were cashing in some trade credits earned through their work for $700 worth of pediatric dental work, plus eyeglasses valued at $223. Because they are members of an exchange, the Bufords did not have to trade dollar for dollar with one individual. They could have bartered their earned trade credits with a restaurant, caterer or even a cheesecake company. (I'll bet you were wondering how I was going to relate all this to food.)

I called N.C.E. and learned that the local chapter is part of a national network. The St. Louis Association currently lists no supermarkets, but had at one time included some. N.C.E. or other bartering exchanges in your area may offer that option. By joining, you might be able to trade some of your personal goods and services for fruit baskets, wedding cakes, a catered dinner party, an evening out at a fine restaurant or just plain groceries.

When a business joins National Commercial Exchange, it is billed a one time membership fee of $500, half of which can be paid in barter. In addition, the purchaser pays a 10% cash commission to the office each time a product or service is received. Sellers call N.C.E. for an authorization number and the buyer's account is credited. Receipts are kept by all parties, including the office. Members receive a detailed monthly

*From *USA Today*, 10/18/90

statement recapping all purchases. There are also renewal fees yearly; each exchange has a different format.

In addition to record-keeping, exchange organizations actively promote participating businesses in a number of ways. N.C.E. in St. Louis mails a monthly newsletter that includes advertising and lists of what members want. If a needed service or business is not already part of N.C.E., the Association tries to enlist one.

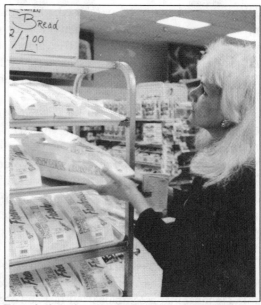

There's little time for baking this week, so Rhonda stocks up on bargain bread.

SHARE

Joining a trade organization may or may not qualify as an important means of saving money on food. But there is another option. Meet SHARE, Self Help and Resource Exchange, headquartered in San Diego, California. SHARE is a non-profit, national, 10 year old program whose primary goal is "to build community by helping people work together to stretch their food budget."

Here's how it works. A community organization — a church, tenants' group or club, for example — fills out an application to become a host organization. This host provides a place where members and people in the neighborhood can register for discounted food packages. Each package is the same within each region, a $30 to $35 value for $13. It always includes six to 10 pounds of meat, four to seven fresh vegetables, two to four fresh fruits, pasta, rice, or cereal, and a few specialty items.

At registration, participants pledge two hours of community service for every package to be purchased. Pledges can be fulfilled through normal church and volunteer activities, or even through helping to package bulk foods at the SHARE warehouse. The host organization tallies the number of packages requested, places an order with local SHARE headquarters, and sends a team of volunteers to pick up and bring back the food.

SHARE doesn't quite fit into a "bartering" or "cooperative" category. The program is open to everyone who is commited to consistent community participation, so in a sense, a discounted food package is bartered for volunteer work. SHARE's volume-buying power gives it some of the advantages of — though little similarity to — a cooperative.

SHARE is rapidly expanding and may be in your area now or in the near future. To find a nearby location, see Resources.

GET ORGANIZED

Have you ever stood in your kitchen at 4:45 p.m., dismally scanning the shelves for ideas for dinner? That's me sometimes, hoping for a miracle meal that assembles itself fast and easily. It doesn't happen!

Meal Plan

That's why I was fascinated by a strategy proposed by Adrianne Ferree of *The Frugal Times*. Adrianne writes out a menu for the month, 30 days' worth of meals at a time. Breakfast, lunch and dinner are included. Favorite meals are repeated as often as desired. Allowances are made for leftovers, new recipes and times for eating out.

Recently I gave Adrianne's system a try. I pulled out an old calendar and jotted down 30 flexible entries. Some were purposefully vague, like "stew" and "chicken dish." My idea was to loosely structure our meals, yet still take advantage of supermarket sales, especially on meat. It's surprising how much more in control I felt, knowing in advance what I planned to serve.

Do Once-a-Month Cooking

Adrianne prepares many of the meals on her monthly list in a single day. I've learned that others do, too. Take Mimi Wilson and Mary Beth Lagerborg, for instance: these women have written a comprehensive book called *Once-a-Month Cooking (A Time-Saving, Budget-Stretching Plan to Prepare Delicious Meals)*. Mimi and Mary Beth not only cook all at once, they also do the majority of their monthly grocery shopping on one day.

They explain, "Each entree is partially prepared or cooked and assembled in advance. Then they're put into sealed containers and stored in the freezer. When you're ready to serve a certain meal, all you have to do is thaw it, combine the ingredients, and cook the entree. And all that time-consuming preparation and cleanup is done at one time."

To help poor struggling cooks like me, Mimi and Mary Beth provide detailed shopping lists and menu plans. By using their system, they promise several benefits: "...after we've prepared a month or two weeks of meals, we don't have to fall back on less-nutritious, quick-fix foods or the more costly restaurant meals.... You can also save more money — and lots of time — when you make fewer trips to the store. Once you have your entrees in the freezer, you've done a major portion of your food preparation for the month."

The only disadvantage I can see to marathon cooking is the cash outlay required. When one is shopping for ingredients for very specific meals, it is much more difficult to utilize store sales. I think I come out ahead by serving flexible menus that make good use of specials. Still, the system seems worth considering. (See Resources under *Once-a-Month Cooking* and *Dinner's In the Freezer*.)

Use Leftovers

Menu-planning is one part of good organization. Another, equally important, is wise use of leftovers. Rule #1 is to keep a tight inventory, either mental or written, of foods on hand in the freezer, cupboard and refrigerator. Here are some ideas for using leftovers.

♦ Breads of all kinds: Freeze until you have a bag full. Make stuffing, garlic breadsticks, bread pudding, bread crumbs or croutons.

♦ Fruits: use in Jell-o, popsicles or Frozen Fruit Delight (see Recipes). Ripe bananas work well in banana bread or cookies.

♦ Leftover turkey: make soup, pot pie or enchiladas.

♦ Vegetables: chop or puree and add to ground meat dishes, or store in a freezer "soup pot," ready to simmer when you have a pot's worth.

◆ A variety of leftovers: serve for lunches or snacks. Or make a buffet night where you serve dabs of this and that along with a special dessert.

Most of the above ideas are mine, and I must admit I've been pretty proud of my expertise in thinking of them. Then I discovered *The Use-It-Up Cookbook (A Guide for Minimizing Food Waste)* by Lois Carlson Willand. Now this is a truly comprehensive treatment of leftovers! Included are 190 pages of recipes and good advice, a reheating time chart, storage guide for perishable foods, detailed index and much more. Name just about any food you can think of, and you can find it here, along with dozens of ways to creatively recycle it. Lois says her cookbook is available at some libraries, so check there first. If not, it is certainly worth the price. See Resources.

MAKE OR COOK YOUR OWN

In Chapter Two, I listed several ways to save money when buying specific foods at the store. Another alternative is to save money when *preparing* these same foods. Then, if you buy an item cheaply and also cut some of the preparation costs, your savings are doubled.

Meats and Other Proteins

Let's say, for example, that you've just bought a whole chicken for 39 cents a pound. To save even more, you can dish up small helpings, or stretch a few ounces a long way in a casserole, ethnic dish or hearty soup.

Perhaps you can substitute more vegetarian dishes in your diet and make even better use of your food dollars. A variety of healthy foods (from USDA's food pyramid or the basic four food groups) will add up to plenty of complete proteins in the course of a day, even without meat. Jackie Iglehart, editor of *The Penny Pincher,* prepares several dishes from cooked beans; she buys 25 pound bags of dry pintos from a food co-op for 41 cents a pound. By teaming beans, homemade breads, grains such as brown rice, several vegetables and fruits, the Igleharts are able to serve low-cost, protein-rich meals for 25 to 50 cents per person.

Cheaper meat tastes better when prepared carefully. Marinades and tenderizers improve both quality and texture, and they need not be expensive. Mary Ellen, in *Mary Ellen's Helpful Hints*, suggests rubbing a roast with a marinade of vinegar and oil, then letting it stand in the refrigerator for two hours before baking.

I often cook meat with a Crock-Pot; eight hours yields fall-off-the-bone texture, and every tidbit is used. Pressure cookers are another option, especially when preparing tougher meats. Some cuts, like beef brisket, can be covered with water in a Dutch oven, simmered for three or four hours until tender, and sliced thinly across the grain.

Dairy Foods

Before you shop the dairy aisle, be aware that there are a number of substitutions you can make at home to save money. Dry milk is often — not always — less costly than liquid, especially if you follow directions carefully and don't load up the drink with extra powder. For great, cheap cocoa, mix a teaspoon of plain cocoa and a little sugar or sweetener with 1/2 cup very hot water, blending well. Add 2/3 cup dry milk powder and enough icy cold water to make three cups of delicious chocolate milk or cocoa.

Use dry milk powder to make your own sweetened condensed milk. Create homemade, low-fat sour cream in the blender. Another dairy substitute, one for whipped topping, can also be created from scratch. See pages 98 and 99 for the recipes.

We have saved more than $1.00 a week by switching from soft margarine to stick margarine. Granted, $1.00 doesn't seem like much until you realize it's 1/50th of our budget! And did you know you can make your own soft margarine, one that is lower in fat than the regular version? Using a beater, thoroughly blend skim milk into a pound of margarine. You'll have to experiment to see what works best for you, but I've found that I can add almost a cup of milk per four sticks.

You can also create your own yogurt. Several years ago a neighbor shared with us several large boxes of nonfat milk powder; she received them free and never used them. When I picked up a yogurt maker for $1 at a garage sale, we began churning out yogurt for nothing! The process is very easy with a machine; I simply follow the manufacturer's directions. If you have access to low-cost milk it may be worth your while. See Recipes, page 101, for yogurt made in the oven.

Breads, Grains, Pasta, Cereals

Save on breads, grains and cereals by cooking a quick, nutritious breakfast. In Donna McKenna's booklet, *The $30 a Week Grocery Budget*, she lists the following mainstays for breakfast at her house: hot cereals, fried cornmeal mush, oatmeal, Cream of Wheat, French toast, muffins, pancakes, waffles, and donuts made by frying refrigerator biscuits. Any of these options is much cheaper than cold cereal with milk.

Jackie Iglehart, publisher of *The Penny Pincher*, recommends using a breadmaker. She claims that, even with an initial outlay of $234, her machine paid for itself in a few months and now saves her $500 a year. A baker sells flour and yeast at cost to Jackie, enabling her to produce a loaf of homemade bread for 15 cents! If you're interested in learning more, see Resources.

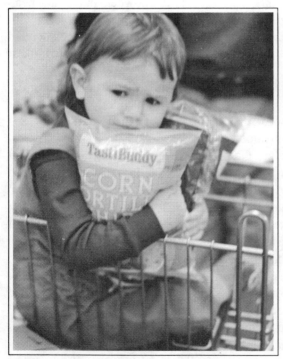

Little Mary can't reach for items on the shelf when her hands are already occupied!

Another option is to keep a big batch of yeast bread dough in your refrigerator. *More-with-Less Cookbook* says any dough with at least one tablespoon sugar per cup of flour can be stored chilled for up to three days. Grease the top of the kneaded dough and cover with plastic, then a damp cloth, before refrigerating. Punch down as needed. Bring dough to room temperature two hours before baking, and let it rise until doubled, about one and a half to two hours. Bake as usual.

To cut baking costs, try substituting margarine for oil or cutting the amount of oil in half. Cater to recipes that feature cheaper whole grains, such as oatmeal bread instead of whole wheat bread. Sometimes applesauce or white syrup can be used in place of shortening (*Fat-Free Indulgences*, listed in Resources, tells you how in several different recipes). Leave out nuts if they are prohibitively expensive, or use a cheaper variety. Try to bake several items at once; I like to brown granola at the same time I'm preparing cakes, and save on energy costs.

Other Foods
Baby Food and Formula

Nurse if you possibly can, and for as long as you can. You can't beat the cost, convenience or nutrition! La Leche League International will be glad to answer any questions you may have on breastfeeding, and there's no obligation or fee. See Resources.

When your infant is ready for more solid food, check the local library for books on making your own baby food. To tell you the truth, my children went from nursing full time to slightly-bland, mashed-up table food. I used to puree leftovers and freeze them in ice cube trays, then microwave what I needed at the last minute. Most of the time my babies ate right along with us. (Of course, caution must be taken: no honey for children under a year old, for example, and no nuts. Popcorn, hot dogs and grapes must be cut into miniscule pieces. Ask your pediatrician.)

Drinks

We make orange juice from frozen concentrate as Aldi's brand is much cheaper than ready-made; compare prices in your area for the best buy. If the children have reached their daily quota of milk products, I reduce the sugar and serve off-brand Kool-aid, one cup per person. We drink water in the car when we're out and about, between meals and as "seconds" at meals.

The Penny Pincher contains a recipe for homemade seltzer in issue #7; see Resources.

Here's an idea for stretching coffee from Larry Roth of *Living Cheap News*; he takes the used grinds from a Mr. Coffee-type coffee maker, lets them cool, refrigerates, then adds new coffee to the existing grounds. "I use three and a half spoons for the first pot," he says, "and, for each subsequent pot, I add two and a half spoons until the filter is full. I then throw it all out and start over." Larry says he can't tell any difference in the taste. For a gourmet flavor, try adding a pinch of salt, a little vanilla or some cinnamon.

Popsicles

This is a standard snack for us, especially in the summertime. I picked up two Tupperware mold sets at yard sales, and made my money back in two weeks. Usually I freeze fruit juice. But other ambitious parents I know have tried gelatin, pudding, yogurt, Kool-aid and just about anything else on hand.

Salad Dressings

I've found homemade dressings and croutons team up to make a delicious, inexpensive salad. See Recipes, pages 86, 100 and 101.

Sauces and Soups

Again, make your own. *More-with-Less Cookbook* says a good basic white sauce, found in nearly every recipe book, takes about five minutes. From the parent recipe you can create cheese sauce, gravy and a number of variations, none of them necessarily high in fat or calories See Recipes, pages 75 and 83.

Broth is another commodity that's cheap and simple: add a little extra water to the roast or chicken you're baking, collect the liquid when you're finished and skim off the extra fat. If you refrigerate the broth, fat solidifies at the top and is easily removed. I freeze excess broth and always have a supply on hand. Use it in homemade gravies, or start a soup pot in the freezer; when there's enough liquid, vegetables and meat, you're ready to simmer up a stew.

Seasonings

You may want to purchase spices at discount or drug stores, or in bulk from a co-op, warehouse or health food store, where they are almost always cheaper. But do try the recipe for taco seasoning in Recipes, page 76.

Syrup

Make your own imitation maple syrup and save at least 75% over store cost. Or try my delicious pancakes: they're so moist they taste just fine with a simple dusting of powdered sugar. See Recipes, page 93.

GARDEN

We planted our first real garden this year, and the whole experience was a dismal one. While the neighbors' tomato plants yielded dozens of firm, delicious fruit, our scraggly vines produced about ten. And a woodchuck from the nearby woods ate half of them. Our beans were so badly chewed we didn't get a single pod. Obviously we have much to learn about gardening.

Extension Services

Thankfully, there is help for people like me. I called the Missouri Botanical Gardens, and was referred to our land grant university's extension service (sometimes called county extension service). Off-campus faculty translate the teaching and research of the university into workable knowledge for people of the state. When I spoke with John Whelan, Horticulture Specialist at the University of Missouri, I was impressed with the scope of the program.

John sent me a listing of sample publications, most of them free or costing 25 to 50 cents each, on topics as varied as a vegetable planting calendar, mulching, soil preparation, how to grow specific fruits and vegetables, making your own compost bins and dozens more. Some of the pamphlets are very specific, such as *Home Production of Black Walnuts and Nut Meats*. You can also read about canning, freezing and food preservation.

In short, your nearby university (county) extension service should have just about everything you need to know regarding gardening and related topics. If you are unsure how to find such a program, refer to the book *Ortho Problem Solver*, available at many home and garden centers. One section contains a listing of every extension service, with phone numbers and addresses, in the United States.

Gardening Books

A trip to the library can supply you with plenty of reading material. Look for gardening magazines or classics, like *Crockett's Victory Gardens* (Little, Brown & Co.). *Square Foot Gardening* (Rodale Press), tells you how to make the most of your garden space and conserve water and labor at the same time. *Gardening By Mail* (Houghton Mifflin Co.) is a sourcebook that lists what's available to you through mail order, and can be found in many libraries' reference departments.

Gardening centers and nurseries may also feature good books. *All About Vegetables*, an Ortho publication, was recommended to me by horticulturists at the Botanical Gardens. Very specific sources like this one, as well as organic gardening magazines, are likely to be found at home and garden centers. Salespeople are usually knowledgeable and truly willing to help, and you can take advantage of their expertise.

Garden Clubs and Associations

Perhaps you would enjoy a more cooperative effort in your gardening. If so, local garden clubs may be the answer. St. Louis boasts the national headquarters of the National Council of State Garden Clubs. With chapters in all 50 states and another in the District of Columbia, over 275,000 members work together on a number of different projects, vegetable gardening included. Study courses are offered to members. *The National Gardener* magazine, leadership training, flower shows, a scholarship fund and environmental activism are only a few of the many benefits available. To locate a chapter near you, see Resources.

Another option is sharing a community garden space. Many cities nationwide are reclaiming vacant lots and planting vegetable gardens. Write to the American Community Gardening Association to learn about opportunities in your area (see Resources).

So far I haven't found an answer to my "critters in the garden" problem, but I am hopeful. With these kinds of resources available, even I may be able to manage a productive garden next year.

GLEAN

There is much free and low-cost food available, and often it's only a matter of finding and gleaning it.

For example, my sister-in-law Joan has worked out a deal with a local supermarket. The produce department boxes up damaged produce and calls Joan, who picks it up for free. I have not been able to locate a store in my area that will do this, but it may be worth your while to call nearby produce managers and at least ask. The last time Joan visited us, she brought along three crates of cucumbers and a huge box of all sorts of fruits, including strawberries, as a gift. And she still had plenty left over for her own family.

Sometimes orchards or farmers will let you pick "seconds" for free or little cost. A major vegetable company owns fields near my home town and, after harvest, allows anyone interested to glean leftover potatoes or green beans. A family friend, Eunice Welker, used to pick a year's worth of free beans and can 100 quarts or more each summer. Eunice says she has salvaged vegetables from other fields as well, even when on vacation. She checks at local grain elevators to learn harvest days, or simply stops to ask a farmer's permission to glean.

Pass the word around your neighborhood that you'd be glad to take — and give — surplus food. One friend and I occasionally trade leftovers: her family tires of the big roast they cooked on Sunday, and trades meat for a loaf of my homemade bread. When a neighbor moved, leaving behind her refrigerator contents, another friend gathered up the goods and divided them with me. Last summer we shared extra vegetables from my sister-in-law with our neighbors. Gleaning is contagious! And in this way it really is possible to obtain free groceries.

If you plan ahead, you may be able to stock up on inexpensive produce in the summertime. Farmers markets abound in both big cities and rural areas. Downtown St. Louis, for example, boasts a huge gathering of both buyers and sellers at Soulard Market. Go late in the selling day, and preferably on the last selling day of the week, for some spectacular buys. You may walk away with boxes full of fruits and vegetables for practically nothing. Also check out orchards and pick-your-own places, where fruits and vegetables are routinely cheap and sometimes, late in the season, *very* cheap.

Keep your eyes open for salvageable food that's going to waste. I've always loved to run and walk, and used to make it a point to try different routes. One autumn day I noticed an apple tree laden with fruit, much of it on the ground on a nice suburban lawn. Several more pass-bys confirmed that no one was picking the apples. Later that week, I stopped and asked the owner: would he mind if I cleaned up his yard in exchange for apples? He was delighted.

My two little boys and I made numerous trips to that man's backyard. We collected so many apples that I made several batches of applesauce and gave some away as Christmas presents. I sold dozens of bags of fruit to fellow workers. And we had enough apples, stored in a cool closet and eating at least four a day, to last us into January.

Another autumn, I was able to locate a pear tree and glean pears from a busy owner. I have also harvested several pounds of free hickory nuts. The food is there for those who are looking for it.

BENEFIT FROM GOVERNMENT PROGRAMS

Your taxes help support a number of different food programs, and you may need to take advantage of some of them when times are exceptionally hard. Your first step should be a call to the U.S. Department of Agriculture's Food and Nutrition Service. You can find their local number in the blue pages of your phone book.

USDA's Food and Nutrition Service (FNS) provides these services (from Program Fact Sheet, March 1991, FNS):

Food Stamps

Food stamps help low-income families buy more food than their limited budgets allow. The amount of stamps each household receives is based on family size and monthly income.

Food Distribution Programs

FNS distributes food commodities to several different programs, including those in schools, at feeding sites for the elderly, summer camps, Indian reservations and more. An Emergency Food Assistance Program provides surplus commodities as needed.

WIC Program

The Special Supplemental Food Program for Women, Infants and Children (WIC) provides specific foods and nutrition education to pregnant, postpartum and breastfeeding women, infants and children to age five.

Commodity Supplemental Food Program

This program supplies nutritious foods as a diet supplement for low-income pregnant, postpartum or breastfeeding women, infants and children under age six. Participants receive packages of commodity foods. Some states operate a supplemental food program for the elderly as well.

National School Lunch Program

Operating since 1946, school lunches are currently served to over 24 million students daily. Schools receive USDA food commodities and nutrition education.

School Breakfast Program

Breakfast is served at school to students who arrive without a morning meal. Institutions are reimbursed on the basis of meals served at cost, reduced price or free.

Child and Adult Care Food Program

Although similar to the other school food programs, this one operates year-round and provides up to two meals and one snack per day. Family day care homes can receive assistance under some circumstances. Participating adult-care centers serve the disabled and elderly.

Summer Food Service Program

Meals are provided to children during extended summer vacations. The program is operated in areas where at least one-half of the children would qualify for free or reduced-price meals.

Special Milk Program

This program offers cash reimbursement for milk served to children in public and private non-profit schools, high school grades or under, and in some child care institutitons, provided they do not also participate in other federal meal service programs.

Nutrition Education and Training Program

Funds are granted to the states for nutrition education of children and inservice training of teachers and food service personnel. USDA hopes to educate consumers on the relationship between good nutrition and health.

If you think you or your family may qualify for any of these services, Food and Nutrition Service will supply more information. The government will also answer your questions on nutrition; call USDA's Human Nutrition Information Service, Public Information Office (see Resources).

EAT SENSIBLY

Sounds pretty obvious, doesn't it? Yet it suddenly struck me, in speaking recently with a friend, that I don't always eat sensibly. My friend Candace constantly monitors the fat in her family's diet; I do not. Candace rarely serves desserts; I do, and often. Reducing both fat and sugar in my meal planning is a way to eat well *and* save money.

There is also the option of eating less, cutting down on calories as well as costs. I like the advice given by Melodie and Ron Moore in their newsletter, *Skinflint News.* Here's a condensation of their article, "Lose Pounds Not $:"

- Make your own diet meals by saving a variety of healthy leftovers in containers in the freezer, then reheating.

- Cook extra meat and slice for a delicious diet lunch. Not only is the flavor much better, but you will also avoid the high-fat content of most packaged lunch meats.

- If you're craving sweets, have a small portion of a homemade brownie instead of buying those expensive "diet" frozen brownies.

- Eat plenty of fresh, seasonal fruit and vegetables.

- Take low-calorie snacks to work with you rather than facing the temptation of the vending machine.

- Drink lots of water or iced tea. For those who crave diet sodas, buy cans by the case.

- Exercise to cut your appetite.

- Consider forming or joining a support group rather than a costly weight loss clinic.

- Think of your dieting as a long term health benefit rather than a short term deprivation. You will be avoiding high-cost health problems brought on by extra weight.

Are you amazed, as I was, to learn of so many ways to save money on groceries? Use some or all of these strategies — wherever you live, whatever your circumstances — and you really *can* eat well for $50 a week.

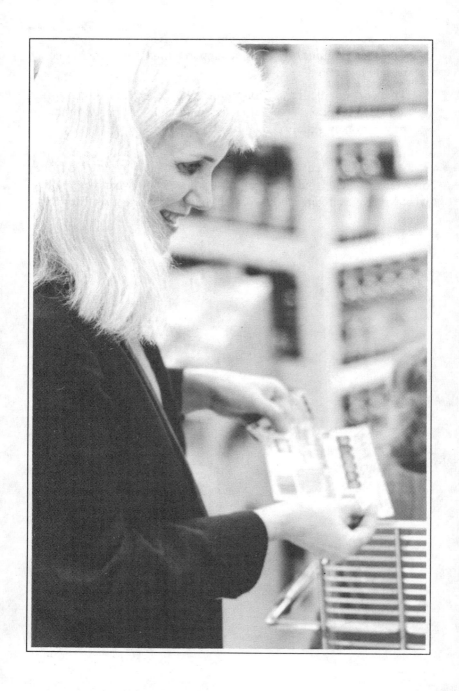

How Do I Ever Manage
To Do All This?

*N*ow that you've read several chapters, are you inspired enough to begin cutting back on your grocery bills? Or are you discouraged? Does it all seem too complicated and time-consuming?

Not long ago I attended a meeting where the speaker was supposed to motivate the rest of us to get organized. Unfortunately, just the opposite resulted. We all looked around rather hopelessly at each other, wondering how in the world we could *ever* accomplish what this woman did in a single day.

I hope you don't feel the same way about saving money on food. It does take time and organization. But I guarantee that you can do it, once you find your own system, and save substantially in a relatively painless way.

But in order to demonstrate this a little more clearly, let me paint a hypothetical picture for you. Penny Price will be my make-believe person, the main shopper and meal planner for the Price family. Her husband John and three school-age children — Susan, Steve and Danny — are also involved. Let's say that Penny has read this book and decides it's time to take action. We'll follow her and her family through a year and observe the changes in their lifestyle.

January 2

Penny shops as usual at her preferred store. She carries along a small notebook and jots down prices on stock-up items like flour, sugar, milk, coffee, and bread. Penny takes a little longer than usual to check out store and generic brands and also writes down their cost in her notebook.

January 9

This week, Penny stops by a nearby grocery store, one she seldom frequents simply out of habit. As she records prices in her notebook, she's surprised to find some items significantly cheaper than those at her usual store. She also discovers an out-of-the-way bin where marked-down meat is stored. She learns from the meat manager that surplus cuts are placed in the bin each morning, often at a 50% savings.

January 16

Penny visits a large warehouse store with her price book. Cost-per-ounce signs help her decide whether buying in bulk would really save money. She concludes that some purchases, like dry cereal, cheese and soda, are definitely cheaper at the warehouse, and she resolves to shop there once a month.

January 23

At the breakfast table the morning before shopping, Penny compares two grocery store fliers and notes several items she needs on sale at National. She checks her price book and sees that the "loss leader" foods are a good buy, cheaper than any other prices in the area. She does all her shopping at National this week.

January 30

Penny checks out a meat market just across from the mall, right on her way home from other errands. She speaks with the butcher and gets some good advice on bargain cuts of meat and how to cook them. Penny buys chicken leg quarters on sale, several pounds at a considerable savings. She asks the butcher to wrap the poultry in two-pound packages and freezes all but one package for future use.

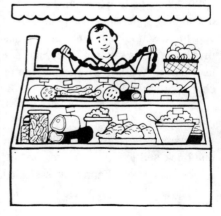

February 6

Susan, eager to be a "good helper" to her mother, clips several coupons from the Sunday paper and arranges them in an envelope alphabetically. As Penny goes through supermarket fliers this week, she matches several sale items with coupons for even greater savings. She plans to shop at Schnucks as they offer the best buys on what she needs, as well as double coupons.

February 13

Penny takes a critical look at the kinds of goods she's been buying and decides to eliminate several convenience foods. This week, she purchases store brand tea bags rather than a six-pack of soda, bulk buy raisins instead of lunch-size packages, and generic toasted oats in place of name brand cereals.

February 20

John and the children sit down together and read through the book *Square Foot Gardening*. A visit to the library provides even more valuable information, including some gardening magazines and *Gardening by Mail*, a resource book on where to order supplies. Once they decide on the garden's layout, Danny and John plan to start seedlings in a warm, sunny corner of their walkout basement.

February 27

The Prices have invited the Aldens for Saturday brunch, and plan a special "theme meal" with pancakes as the main dish. John prepares a huge batch of oatmeal pancakes the night before, first adding bananas, nuts, chocolate chips and bits of cheese to four separate bowls of batter. When the Aldens arrive, a buffet is ready with syrup, honey, fruit sauce, yogurt and ice cream as complements. The two families can't remember ever having so much fun at a company meal!

March 5

Penny finds some intriguing new recipes and decides to give them a try. First she whips up an easy French salad dressing. She makes her own croutons and stuffing mix, using leftover bread ends. She tries a basic white sauce recipe, adding mushrooms, to substitute for canned soup in the chicken casserole she's serving tonight. And she bakes a triple batch of cake from scratch in less time than it takes to put together a single cake mix. Penny's hour in the kitchen saves the Price family about $15.

March 12

John decides to brown bag three times a week instead of eating lunch out. Susan, Steve and Danny begin packing lunchboxes on the same days. John assembles peanut butter and jelly sandwiches, cheese slices, popcorn, carrot sticks with dip, raisins, pretzels, crackers, leftovers of all kinds and homemade cookies. The Prices estimate they can bank at least $20 weekly by bringing their own food from home for noontime meals.

March 19

John starts a new system for making coffee, a necessary expense in the Price household! He mixes used grounds with new ones for a 50% savings. Penny cuts back to two cups of coffee a day and plans to drink more water instead.

March 26

One brisk weekend day, Penny is in the mood for homemade bread. She tries a 90-minute recipe (see Cinnamon Yeast Bread in Recipes) and bakes four loaves. The children help, forming their own smaller dough balls, rolling them out and sprinkling on cinnamon and sugar. Danny loves the taste of hot-out-of-the-oven bread so much that he asks to make it again soon. In a few weeks he is able to turn out loaves from start to finish all by himself.

April 2

Penny visits the warehouse store again after an absence of several weeks. She is a smarter buyer this time around, and doesn't succumb, as she did during her first visit, to the temptations of boxed donuts and ready-made cheesecake. For breakfast the next morning Penny fries refrigerator biscuits (sale-priced last week at 4/$1) and dips her own "donuts" in powdered sugar. She makes a cheesecake from scratch for about $1.50. Between these two items alone she saves more than $8.00 over the warehouse's already low prices.

April 9

Penny and John have made it a point to talk more frequently with Susan, Steve and Danny about nutrition, and so have been both buying and eating healthier foods. When the children arrive home from school now, they often fill up on celery with low-fat cream cheese, peanut butter and crackers, orange juice popsicles, or dry toasted oat cereal mixed with raisins. Fresh fruit has also become a favorite.

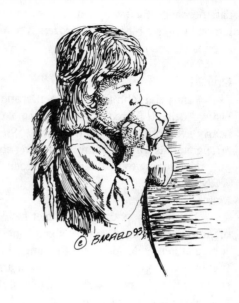

April 16

Penny by now is quite a pro at using up leftovers, and the Prices waste very little food. The freezer holds a large plastic container where leftover bits of meat, vegetables and broth accumulate until there is enough for a kettle of stew. Penny checks the refrigerator and shelves at least twice a week for odds and ends. Those foods that can't be turned into soup are served at Thursday night dinner, smorgasbord-style.

April 23

John goes shopping this week, checking out a new produce stand on his way home from work. The manager is anxious for business and talks with John for a few minutes about seasonal fruit and other bargains. Bananas are on special, six pounds for $1.00. John buys $10.00 worth of fruit, including several bunches of bananas.

April 30

After a week of eating bananas twice a day, the Prices decide to freeze the excess. Some bananas are skewered on popsicle sticks and dipped in caramel sauce, then wrapped in wax paper. The rest are pureed with a little lemon juice in a blender and frozen in two-cup containers, later to be used in banana bread.

May 7

Penny and John sit down together and do some serious meal planning. Using Adrianne Ferree's system, they make a simple listing of 30 meals that nearly everyone in the family enjoys. Steve constructs a chart and helps arrange meals for the month, projecting ahead for days the family will eat out and planning to be flexible as needed.

May 14

The neighbors down the street have joined a commercial exchange organization and tell the Prices about bartering. After careful consideration, John and Penny decide against joining. Instead, they contact several close friends and propose an informal kind of arrangment: any family who has a surplus will try to swap with another family who has a need. Penny agrees in advance to barter garden vegetables for the use of another family's canner.

May 21

The Prices make a joint decision to budget the amount of money spent in eating out together. After a couple of weeks of casually checking out restaurant coupons, they have decided that takeout pizza is their best bet. It's about half the cost of dining at their favorite steakhouse. They'll still splurge

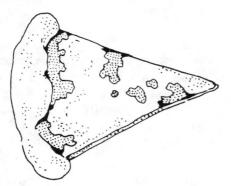

occasionally, of course. But by saving their restaurant money in a piggy bank, they'll soon have the extra cash they need to buy a family membership at the pool this summer.

May 28

Penny and John have gradually made some major changes in their diet, and are a little thinner and more fit than they were six months ago. Everyone now eats less red meat and more beans, rice and pasta; less sugary desserts and more nutritious alternatives. As they've cut their food bill, Penny and John have also cut their cholesterol levels and their weight.

June 4

It's vegetable planting time! One warm Saturday the Prices bring seedlings up from the basement and ready the soil in their garden plot. They barter the use of a neighbor's tiller in exchange for John and Steve restacking the man's disorganized firewood. The Prices are also able to locate fertilizer and some needed tools on sale at a nearby nursery. The garden is planted by dinner time.

June 11

John, head gardener of the family, visits the University of Missouri Extension Service. He wants to get the latest information on "integrated pest management" so the Prices won't have to spend money on — and face health risks from — pesticides. John speaks in person with an expert advisor. He also takes with him some free brochures on ways to maximize vegetable growth, build his own compost pile and have the garden soil tested.

June 18

John, Penny and the children spend a Saturday morning at a pick-your-own strawberry patch. They've come at the end of the season and are able to glean berries at half the usual cost. The family picks enough to have plenty of homemade jam, strawberry desserts and plain good snacking fare.

June 25

Sunday is a perfect summer day, and the Price family decides to spend the afternoon at the zoo. Their usual custom is to eat the food stand's overpriced hot dogs, popcorn and soda. Today they pack a picnic instead. The $15 designated for a late lunch is used to purchase books at the zoo's gift shop.

July 2

Three of the Prices have birthdays this month, and Penny decides to bake the cakes herself. She makes a triple batch of pound cake (see Recipes) and freezes two finished sheet cakes. Next comes a triple batch of frosting and again, two containers are frozen. Penny has already ordered *Baker's Easy Cut-Up Party Cakes* and the birthday boy and girls have decided on designs. Thanks to advance preparation, each cake requires less than 20 minutes for final assembly.

July 9

The garden is growing nicely and the first crop of string beans comes in. The Prices cook a big batch for supper, using a ham bone for flavoring. As other produce ripens over the course of the summer, Penny contacts her friend about the swap they had agreed to earlier: use of a canner in exchange for some vegetables. Now the family will be able to put up several quarts each of beans, peas and tomatoes themselves.

July 16

Penny learns that several church friends are organizing a co-op buying club. She attends an organizational meeting and carefully examines the supplier's catalog. For about an hour's worth of work each month, Penny can buy some products at a real savings, including bulk yeast, spices, cheese and nuts. She joins the co-op.

July 23

John, hungry for something home-baked, rescues pureed bananas and frozen strawberries from the freezer. A couple of hours later he's taking three large, steaming loaves of banana-berry bread from the oven. The Prices gobble down one loaf that night and enjoy generous slices for lunch the next two days.

July 30

Penny's brother and his family are spending the weekend and the Prices intend to entertain them in style. Penny brings out lasagna, home-made French bread and cake from the freezer for Friday night's meal. Saturday features a barbeque with grilled marinated chicken, corn on the cob and fresh garden vegetables. Sunday dinner is turkey with all the trimmings. Penny's brother and sister-in-law enjoy the home-cooked meals, and are convinced their relatives have spent a fortune to feed them. (The Prices don't tell them otherwise!)

August 6

Susan has become so skilled at using coupons that, shopping with her mother, she's able to save more than $7.00 at the store this week. Penny has promised that her daughter can bank any money saved on coupons, so Susan is especially attentive to good deals. She has even set up a coupon exchange box at the library and checks it regularly.

August 13

John has just learned about a new farmers' market in the city, a 30 minute drive from home. Word has it that farmers there sell their goods at tremendous savings toward the end of the day. The Price family makes a trip downtown to check it out. They arrive late afternoon Saturday and, sure enough, come away with two large crates of produce for a fraction of normal supermarket prices.

August 20

Using some of the money they've saved on groceries, the Prices have purchased a used chest-type freezer. Penny has been collecting garage-sale containers all summer and has quite a stockpile. Vegetables and fruits from the farmers' market on Saturday are carefully sorted, processed and frozen. Between the market's produce and their own garden's yield, the Price freezer is nearly full.

August 27

A librarian approaches Susan as she checks her coupon trading box: has she heard about refunding? The librarian locates the name and address of *Refund Express*. Susan sends for a sample copy. She is amazed to receive an 80 page newsprint magazine filled with inspiring stories, numbers to call for free products, and hundreds of ads where swaps can be made for coupons and refund offers. Susan signs up as a subscriber.

September 3

It's taken the Prices eight months, but their weekly grocery bill is now down to about $50. John and Penny's usual routine involves a trip to the warehouse store the first week of each month, where they stock up on lower-cost bulk items. The next three weeks Penny shops at one of two grocery stores, depending on which has the best specials and the best match-up with Susan's coupons. Penny also stops by the meat market occasionally. The produce stand, right on her way to one of the supermarkets, is usually so much cheaper that she often makes a quick run in for fruits and vegetables.

September 10

Steve, riding his bike around the block, has noticed a neighbor's pear tree. Several trips by confirm that no one is picking the fruit. With Penny's approval, Steve leaves a note on the neighbor's door politely requesting that he be allowed to pick the pears. He gets a call the next day from an elderly man who's happy to have his fruit gleaned. Steve stops by one day after school and cleans the man's yard, carefully picking up the grounded pears that are salvageable. (The rotted ones are hauled home to the family compost pile.) Dozens are eaten for snacks. And the rest Steve sells door to door, collecting a tidy sum for his "new bike" fund.

September 17

While out looking for garage sales, Penny notices an obscure day-old bread store and stops to investigate. The prices are excellent. She stocks up on bagels, dinner rolls, hamburger buns and several loaves of whole-grain bread. Donuts are marked three boxes/$1.00 and Penny buys six boxes. Some she freezes and the rest are steamed over a kettle of hot water to almost-fresh quality.

September 24

The Prices have "put out the word" throughout their neighborhood that they will gladly accept any free food or goods, especially those that might otherwise go to waste. Soon friends are calling them: a hunter who has extra venison to share, a gardener who doesn't want to process all of her bumper tomato crop. The Prices graciously follow up with homemade bread loaves as thank-yous.

October 1

Autumn weather has everyone in the mood to pick apples. John, Penny, Susan, Steve and Danny make a day of it at a nearby orchard, gathering over 50 pounds of fruit. They save about 70% compared to normal supermarket prices and have a wonderful time as well. The orchard owner supplies all three children with free small pumpkins as a bonus. Best of all, the whole family enjoys a wagon ride behind the farmer's tractor.

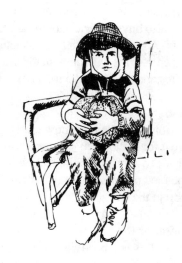

October 8

Penny has just read *Once-a-Month Cooking* and decides to try two weeks' worth of shopping plans and menus. She sets aside a Saturday morning for shopping and a Sunday evening for cooking. The system works very well. Penny is surprised at how much is accomplished in a short time, and soon she has 14 entrees ready in the freezer.

October 15

Penny and the children decide to prepare for Halloween a little early this year. Together, they create an enormous batch of cookie dough and a triple recipe of caramel corn. Steve bags the caramel corn for his school party, and also helps Penny roll out dough and cookie-cut. Susan and Danny frost and decorate little pumpkin-shaped sugar cookies. The children don't mind their chores since the rewards — bites of treats — are definitely worth the bother.

October 22

Susan wants to have a few friends over for dinner and a sleepover. The Prices agree, and set a $10 spending limit. No problem, Susan says. She scans her bulging coupon collection and pulls out several to use at a store offering double savings. She buys bread, deli meat packages, cheese and soda on sale. With her coupons, they're only a fraction of the original cost. Susan also buys generic napkins and plates and glues on handmade autumn motifs. A menu for eight friends includes turkey and cheese sandwiches on buns, corn chips with homemade dip, carrot sticks, pretzels, caramel corn, cookies and soda, all at a total cost of $9.68.

October 29

John and the boys buy a large pumpkin from the produce stand and carve it for Halloween. The seeds are washed, dried and oven-roasted. In a day or two the pumpkin itself will be cut into pieces, cooked and pureed in the food processor. Penny will make a few pies and have plenty left over to pop in the freezer.

November 5

Halloween candy is on sale, so Penny purchases several large bags. She knows from experience that discounted candy bars and M&M's are often cheaper than baking chips. Penny freezes all the goodies in hidden reaches so no one will be overly tempted. Over the next few months she has a large cache of both treats and baking chocolate.

November 12

Thanksgiving is two weeks away and turkeys are on sale at the supermarket. Penny relies on her stockpile of other foods and spends most of the grocery budget on meat. She buys a whole turkey at 39 cents a pound and freezes it. She also invests in extra cranberries, margarine, whipped topping and other sale items.

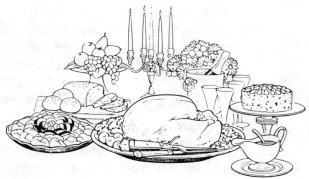

November 19

Steve, the entrepreneur of the family, has found another source of income: nuts. While exploring a family friend's "back 40," he's located an out-of-the-way pecan tree. Steve gets permission to gather over a bushel and spends several hours shelling pecans. Penny and several neighbors buy large containers full of nuts for $5.00 each, still a good savings over store prices. Steve soon has another $35.00 to put in the bank. At this rate he'll have enough money for his new bike by spring.

November 26

As the Prices celebrate Thanksgiving, they are truly thankful for their bountiful harvest of food. Penny has bought a second, fresh turkey and made her own stuffing and gravy. The menu also includes peas and potatoes from the garden. Using some of Steve's pecans, Susan and Danny have baked a banana nut loaf. John's special offering is his own cranberry relish, Penny's, a homemade pumpkin pie. The meal has been a real cooperative effort. But the results are outstanding in both savings and taste.

December 3

Penny and a group of friends meet for an informal potluck at the Prices' house. The discussion turns to the astronomical cost of feeding a family, and Penny shares some of the strategies she's learned in the past year. Three women agree to try an informal swap of Christmas cookies next week in an effort to save both time and money. The Prices, the Aldens and the Fergusons will each bake triple batches of three different recipes, delivering one batch of each to the others' homes.

December 10

John is in the mood for Christmas shopping. Instead of heading for the mall, the family brainstorms some ideas for homemade presents. Danny wants to give his own special yeast bread. Susan decides to make coupon holders, each with 50 coupons filed alphabetically inside. Steve plans to share jars of canned pears, the ones he foraged from a neighbor three months earlier. John and Penny will buy some items, of course. But for friends and co-workers, they decide to give homemade chocolate creams (see Recipes), rosettes and decorated cookies. They estimate a savings of at least $150 over last year, when most of their gifts averaged $10 per person.

December 17

Penny has budgeted ahead, and plans to take advantage of holiday sales. The meat market has just advertised whole hams at half price, so she buys two. Susan is enthusiastically clipping coupons; many more are available now during the holiday season. Between both sales and double coupons, the Prices' grocery bill is less than half of the regular cost of food.

December 24

Penny and John exchange Christmas gifts shortly after the children are in bed for the night. Along with a few romantic offerings, John has also bought a breadmaker for Penny (and the family!). For an investment of about $250, the Prices calculate that their machine will pay for itself in six months. After that they'll have daily fresh-baked loaves for 20 cents each, and with only a few minutes' time invested.

December 31

As the new year rolls in, the Prices make a resolution: to save even more this year than last. They have learned much about ways to conserve the food dollar. Now they'll try their hand at other means of cutting back. Their goal is a family vacation to a ski lodge over the holidays next December. With the money they save, they'll be able to do it.

And so Penny, John, Susan, Steve and Danny live happily ever after. And it *is* a fairy tale, I admit, and real life seldom runs so smoothly. The Prices cut food costs in a very realistic way, one step at a time, one new strategy each week. That's what Michael and I have done, and it works. We actually practice much of what the Prices supposedly tried, and I know of many others who manage to accomplish this and much more. The composite picture is fictional but possible.

The idea of my make-believe story is to inspire you. Wouldn't it be fun to write your own, true story this year?

I Can't Save Money On
Groceries Because...

*T*he story of Penny Price is behind us now, and it's time to face reality! Do you think that, for you and your family, eating well on $50 a week is impossible? You spend a lot more than $50, but you have a good excuse, right? Then let's talk about it. Please fill in the blank below:

"I can't save money on groceries because _____."

Now allow me to anticipate some of your answers, and offer some suggestions.

"I can't save money on groceries because I'm too tired to cook and rely on convenience foods for most of my meals."

- Then marathon-cook on a weekend (or some other time when you're more rested) and make your own convenience foods.

- Try some of the recipes in the next chapter. Many entrees can be prepared in half an hour or less.

- Rely more heavily on time-saving devices — such as a Crock-Pot, breadmaker, pressure cooker or food processor — to make cooking faster.

- Menu plan carefully to allow for quick, easy homemade meals on nights when you know you'll be most tired.

"I can't save money on groceries because I'm on a low-cholesterol diet and have to pay more for special foods."

- Then use the booklet *The New Lean Toward Health* to learn how to calculate the number of grams of fat in the foods you eat, then devise an inexpensive diet with no more than 30% of total calories from fat. See Resources.

- Bulk-buy canola oil, brown rice, dry beans and other healthy foods from a warehouse grocer or co-op.

- Combine double coupons with supermarket sales, and stock up on low-fat versions of margarine, sour cream, cheese and other staples when they're cheapest.

- Think of meat as a side dish, and serve only small portions. Cook more chicken and turkey. Fortunately, both are usually cheaper than beef or pork.

- Learn to eat fish. Buy seafood that is currently in season. Better yet, take up fishing.

- Fill up on fresh fruits and vegetables, purchased in season from supermarket sales, produce stands or farmers' markets.

- Serve beans. *More-with-Less Cookbook* features an entire chapter of bean recipes, some as simple as mashing cooked lentils, forming into patties and broiling like hamburgers.

- Do your own baking, but apply these cho-

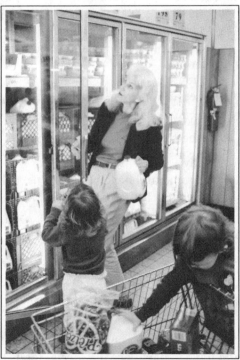

Sometimes powdered milk is cheaper than liquid, but not this week.

lesterol-cutting rules: For cakes and soft-drop cookies, use no more than two tablespoons of fat per cup of flour. For muffins, quick breads and biscuits, use no more than one to two tablespoons of fat per cup of flour (from *The New Lean Toward Health*).

"I can't save money on groceries because I take my young children shopping with me, and I give in when they beg me for expensive treats."

- Then don't give in! (Easier said than done!)

- Talk to your children before you go to the store. Explain that you will be buying only what is on your list.

- Let each child choose one inexpensive treat per visit ahead of time. Any whining or obnoxious behavior forfeits the treat.

- Go to the store at a time when everyone's rested and fed.

- Involve the children in shopping, from fetching cans of corn to going through a pretend purse filled with "real stuff" (just like Mommy uses as the store).

- Take along special toys to keep little hands occupied and attitudes cheerful.

- Play quiet games or read a book during a long wait in the check-out lane.

- Combine firm rules with a pleasant experience, so resistance is minimized the next time.

- Reward well-behaved children with genuine praise. A favorite activity, extra privilege or piece of candy doesn't hurt, either.

"I can't save money on groceries because I do a lot of entertaining."

- Then entertain with home-cooked meals whenever possible. Table-cloths, fresh flowers, candlelight and delicious recipes make the simplest food seem elegant.

- Stick to cheap menus.

- Check out *More-with-Less Cookbook* from the library and read about

Doris Janzen Longacre's "theme meals." Doris focuses on "one nutritious, cheap, but interesting dish," and adds a few simple, complimentary dishes. Her suggestions are intriguing and inexpensive.

- Limit hors d'oeuvres to cheaper varieties. Serve at tables rather than passing on trays.

- Host a potluck. You supply the main dish, dessert, drinks and the house, and guests bring a vegetable, salad and bread.

- Choose an "off-time" for entertaining. Offer only snacks or desserts.

- B.Y.O.B., wine coolers, soda, Kool-aid or juice.

"I can't save money on groceries because I have no car and only have access to an expensive store."

- Then "beat the system" in that store:

- Try to buy only what's on sale, and stock up when you can.

- Ask the store meat manager about marked-down cuts of meat, and deli meat and cheese "ends." A friendly butcher can also offer good advice on bargain meats and ways to tenderize and cook them.

- Talk to the store produce manager about selling slightly-damaged or bruised fruits and vegetables at half price.

- Have your friends and relatives call both the store meat manager and produce manager with the same requests. If enough people ask for discounted foods, supermarkets will usually try to oblige.

- Clip coupons religiously. Visit the store on double-coupon days.

"I can't save money on groceries because we're all big meat eaters, and meat is expensive."

- Then dine on cheaper cuts of meat, like chicken.

- Buy a half or quarter side of beef from the butcher and divide it up, if necessary, with friends.

- Make it a point to only buy meat that's on sale. Stock up when your favorites are cheapest.

- Shop around for a supermarket that sells surplus, marked-down cuts.

- Gradually decrease the portions of meat served in each meal, and supplement with more breads, grains, fruits and vegetables.

"I can't save money on groceries because my children will only eat expensive, highly processed foods."

- Then introduce nutritious alternatives, one at a time, while gradually phasing out the junk. Find a healthy food, like grapes or bananas, that a child really likes, and serve it frequently.

- Begin to substitute raisins for candy, air-popped popcorn for potato chips, and homemade yogurt popsicles for ice cream bars.

- Remember that children go through phases. What they don't like today may become a favorite food tomorrow. Keep reintroducing small portions.

- Involve your children in cooking. When we checked out a "Super-heroes" cookbook from the library, Eric could hardly wait to try — and eat — some nutritious recipes. See Resources, *DC Super Heroes Super Healthy Cookbook*.

- Serve food in a way that's attractive to children. Lisa never liked mashed potatoes until Dad ladled gravy in the middle and called his creation a swimming pool.

- Use "props" to make good food more appealing. Children who don't like milk may drink it from a special thermos or a "grown-up" glass with a special straw. Colorful plates and napkins help, too.

- Avoid food fights by giving children some choices. You can frame the question as "Would you rather eat your peas or banana bread first?" instead of threatening, "If you don't eat those peas right now you're in time-out for an hour!" (I've been foolish enough to say something like this last remark, and know how poorly it works!)

- Don't get into the habit of preparing whatever the child wants, especially if it's always different from the rest of the family's dinner. (There are exceptions to this, especially when you're dealing with a toddler on a temporary "food jag" who will only tolerate jelly sandwiches and applesauce.) Make a comment like, "I'm sorry you don't care for the meatloaf, but this is what we're eating tonight. Would you like to help me prepare one of your favorite meals tomorrow night?"

- Offer no unhealthy alternatives. My children learned to drink water because, one summer, I simply told them that if they were thirsty between meals, they could have all the ice water they wanted. Now they help themselves to the pitcher in the refrigerator several times a day.

- Read and talk about nutrition so your children understand why you're changing their eating habits. Mine were fascinated by the lessons learned from *The Berenstain Bears and Too Much Junk Food:* soon afterward, Christian wanted "crunchy carrot sticks" every day, sometimes several times a day.

- Practice what you preach.

"I can't save money on groceries because I can't be bothered with going to more than one grocery store."

- Then go to one, once a month, and do most of your shopping at a single time. Each week's grocery list should then be much smaller, and making a quick, weekly stop to your regular supermarket a manageable trip.

- "Beat the system" in the one store of your choice in order to maximize your savings there. (See three excuses back for details.)

- Join a cooperative.

- Buy all your meat for the month one week, all your canned and long-term supplies the next week, all your freezeable breads the next, most of your produce the next...you get the idea.

"I can't save money on groceries because I eat only natural, organic, healthy foods."

- Then grow your own, as much as possible, and freeze the excess. Your university (county) extension agent will be glad to show you how to garden organically.

- Buy through a co-op rather than a health food store. If there is currently no co-op in your area, contact the nearest food warehouse for information on how to organize one. See Resources, U.S. Cooperative Food Warehouses.

- Purchase meat and produce directly from farmers you know and trust.

- Glean as much as possible.

- Call a local bartering exchange to find out if joining an exchange might enable you to trade with an organic foods supplier. See Resources, Organizations and More.

- Pick your own fruit and vegetables. Stock up in the summertime, particularly on foods that store well, like apples.

"I can't save money on groceries because I end up buying so many extra treats for birthdays and holidays."

- Then set a budget for birthdays and holidays and stick to it.

- Use your creativity — rather than your pocketbook — to

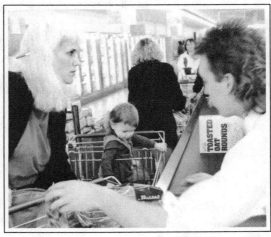

Rhonda checks to see if she's below her $50 limit .

71

make celebrations special. Buy a copy of *Baker's Easy Cut-Up Party Cakes,* for example, to learn how to assemble sensational cakes for next to nothing. See Resources.

- Stock up on food for birthday parties by purchasing ice cream, soda and other treats on sale, using double coupons, if possible. Plan ahead.

- Bulk buy candy as party favors. Package it yourself.

- Understand, when dealing with children, that giving them everything money can buy is fulfilling a want, not a need.

- Compromise. Offer alternatives, such as a sleepover with VCR movies and homemade caramel corn, instead of a pizza party for 20. Is your child willing to finance an expensive party from his own savings?

- Give homemade gifts of food at Christmas time. See any of the December issues of thrift newsletters (listed in Resources) for excellent, low-cost ideas.

"I can't save money on groceries because I don't see any need to do so."

- Then calculate how much you're spending on food right now. If your current weekly average is $100, and you cut back to $50, that's more than a $200 monthly savings. (You can also think of it as $200 of tax-free income.) Is there anything else on which you would rather be spending this money?

"I can't save money on groceries because I just plain don't want to."

- Then.....well, sorry. I don't have an answer for that one!

6

Recipes

*B*efore plunging right into actual recipes, I must warn you about something I said in the beginning: I am not an outstanding cook. My purpose in including this chapter is certainly not to try and impress you with my culinary skills. Rather, I could imagine someone writing and saying something like, "You can't *really* make a cake in five minutes, can you? How do you do that?" Hopefully the following recipes will answer some of your questions in advance.

Many of these may almost seem an insult to advanced cooks. Doesn't everybody know how to make tuna salad, for heaven's sake? I used to think so, until meeting several individuals who had no idea how to do anything in the kitchen other than heat up a microwave dinner. So please bear in mind that some of the recipes are definitely geared toward beginners.

There are also some glaring omissions. We eat nearly all of our fruits and vegetables plain and/or fresh, and so there are no "Vegetables" or "Salads" sections here. The dishes included in this chapter are only ones that I personally prepare. The "Meats and Main Dishes" recipes are designed to be used with any one of several differents kinds of meats; this is a real plus when you're buying whatever is on sale.

At any rate, here are several recipes that have been helpful to me as I've learned to eat well for $50 a week.

MEATS AND MAIN DISHES

CHICKEN IN BARBEQUE SAUCE
Serves 6-8

Mix barbeque sauce together in a saucepan:

       1/2 cup chopped onion
       1/2 cup ketchup
       1/2 cup sugar
       2 tsp. Worcestershire sauce
       Dash of pepper

Cook over low heat for three minutes. Set aside. Add enough oil to a frying pan to cover the bottom of the pan. Brown chicken pieces of your choice in hot oil. Drain chicken on paper towels. Place in large, greased casserole dish. Cover with generous amounts of barbeque sauce. Bake in a 350 degree oven for an hour or until tender.
Variations: Use barbeque sauce on pork, beef, turkey or any other meat. Eliminate the frying and bake meat in a Crock-Pot or in the oven.
Tips: Cook vegetables in the oven along with the meat, preferably on a layer below it in the same pan.

CHILI
Serves 6-8

Combine in a large metal saucepan:

       2 15-ounce cans red beans, liquid included
       1 15-ounce can kidney beans, liquid included
       1 large chopped onion
       1 finely chopped green pepper
       1/4 cup sugar
       2 tsp. salt
       Chili powder to taste
       Garlic powder to taste

Simmer for one to two hours, until flavors are well blended.
Serve topped with cheese and croutons.
Variations: Add leftover meat of your choice. Drain liquid from beans and substitute one large can tomato or vegetable juice. Use canned tomatoes and extra seasoning in place of bean liquid. Substitute dry beans in place of canned beans for a better value; see package directions.
Tips: Cook in a Crock-Pot for 8 hours or more; flavor improves with longer simmering time.

CHUCK ROAST WITH VEGETABLES AND GRAVY
Serves 6-8

Preheat oven to 350 degrees.
Place in a large ovenproof pan or Dutch oven:

    3 to 4 pounds chuck roast
    4 potatoes, peeled and diced
    4 carrots, peeled and diced
    2 onions, cut into wedges
    2 cups water

Sprinkle 1 envelope dry onion soup mix over all.
Bake for 2 1/2 to 3 hours, depending on the size of the roast, or until vegetables are tender and meat separates easily with a fork. Remove from oven. Drain drippings from the larger pan into a smaller saucepan. Return meat and vegetables to the oven to keep warm. Skim fat from the drippings.

Gravy
With tightly fitting lid on plastic bowl, shake together until smooth:

    2 Tbsp. cornstarch
    1 cup water
    1 to 2 Tbsp. soy sauce
    Garlic powder, salt and pepper to taste

Add to drippings. Cook and stir constantly over medium heat until liquid thickens and boils. Boil gently for one minute, stirring constantly. Serve immediately with roast and vegetables.
Variations: Cook chicken, pork or beef in a barbeque sauce. Add any in-season vegetables you like.
Tips: If I'm in a hurry I turn up the oven temperature to 375 degrees and add extra water. If time is not important, I sometimes use the Crock-Pot. Crocking is especially good for tough cuts, as eight hours yields very tender, fall-off-the-bone meat. To cut fat, make gravy without drippings and add extra seasonings to taste. Serve small portions of meat and fill up with vegetables.

ENCHILADAS
Serves 4-6

Brown in a frying pan:
>1 pound ground beef
>1 medium onion, chopped

Drain grease. Add:
>1 cup water
>1 package taco seasoning mix

Set aside. Shred several cups of lettuce into one bowl. Grate a few ounces of your favorite cheese into another. Heat one package of flour or corn tortillas in the oven or microwave according to package directions. Assemble on tortillas: cheese, hot meat mixture, lettuce. Fold bottom one-fourth of tortilla horizontally toward the top. Roll rest of tortilla vertically into a cylinder. Secure with toothpicks.

Variations: We usually assemble the enchiladas one at a time at the table. But sometimes I prepare several in advance, line them in a cake pan, spread a thin row of salsa and cheese on top, and bake for 10 minutes in a 400 degree oven. Any meat or bean mixture will substitute for ground beef, but more seasoning is required for chicken, turkey or dried beans. I sometimes add leftover vegetables. Make your own taco seasoning mix, below.

Tips: Tortillas can be made by hand but the process takes time. For a very similar taste, fry the store-bought version in a little oil. This dish is especially quick if the ground beef and onion mixture has been prepared in advance and frozen.

Taco Seasoning Mix
Combine:
>2 tsp. chili powder
>2 tsp. dried parsley flakes
>1 1/2 tsp. cumin
>1 tsp. paprika
>1 tsp. onion salt
>1/2 tsp. oregano
>1/2 tsp. garlic powder

This recipe is equivalent to a 1 1/4 ounce package of store bought seasoning mix, and cheaper, especially if you buy spices in bulk.

HASHBROWNS
Serves 6-8

Cook in the microwave until slightly done but still firm:
        6 large potatoes (I prefer red), peeled
Grate potatoes into a large bowl, and add:
        1 large onion, grated
Heat in a large frying pan:
        1/2 cup oil

Mix potatoes and onions thoroughly and place mixture in hot pan. Cover. Cook over medium heat for about 15 minutes, or until crispy and brown. Turn. Cook another ten minutes. Add salt and pepper as desired.
Variations: Add meat to potato mixture if you like. For a buttery taste, fry in margarine instead of oil. Do not use diet margarine, as potatoes will stick to the pan and tend to burn.
Tips: Serve with sour cream, ketchup or barbeque sauce.

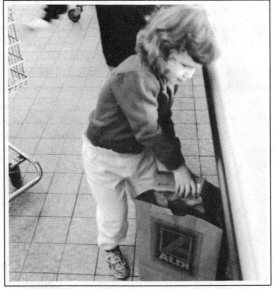

Lisa helps bag groceries. Involving the children makes a shopping trip both faster and more pleasant.

LASAGNA
Serves 14-16

Brown in a large frying pan:
> 1 1/2 pounds ground beef
> 1 large onion, chopped finely

Add and simmer for one hour:
> 2 15-ounce cans tomatoes
> 3 8-ounce cans tomato sauce
> 1/2 cup sugar
> 1 Tbsp. Worcestershire sauce
> 2 Tbsp. Italian seasoning

Meanwhile, in a separate bowl, combine:
> 1 pound small-curd cottage cheese
> 3 eggs
> 1/2 cup Parmesan cheese

Prepare one large package lasagna noodles according to directions. Set aside. Grate and set aside 1 pound mozzarella cheese. Grease two large cake pans. Layer cooked noodles, cottage cheese mixture, mozzarella cheese, tomato sauce, first in one pan, then the other. Bake at 400 degrees for 45 minutes. Let stand for 10 minutes before serving.

Variations: Substitute your favorite spaghetti sauce for the tomato sauce mixture. Skip cooking the noodles, but make sure dry noodles are thoroughly covered with sauce; add a little extra water, then bake the dish at a slightly lower temperature, and a little longer than usual.

Tips: This recipe is expensive to make, but produces quite a lot of a very filling entree. It freezes well and actually improves in flavor after a few days in the refrigerator. I often add more diced vegetables and decrease the amount of meat.

LUNCH MEAT

To make the children's lunches a little more interesting, here are some ideas: Place one thin slice of cheese on one thin slice of lunch meat. Roll up and secure with a toothpick. • Cut lunch meat into small squares. Serve with cheese squares, crackers, a little margarine and other fixings to make your own mini-"sandwiches." • Arrange one slice of lunch meat and one thin slice of cheese on one slice of bread. Supply pickles, olives, carrots sticks, etc. Let the children create "faces" on their sandwiches before eating them. • Serve ham cubes, cheese cubes and chunk pineapple on toothpicks for do-it-yourself shish-kebabs. •Roll a thin slice of meat and a thin slice of cheese inside a flour tortilla.

Tips: I seldom buy prepared lunch meats — like bologna — because of the high fat content. Instead, I wait until a good quality ham is on sale and ask the butcher to slice it very thinly: the meat is delicious and much better for you. We also serve diced turkey.

MEATLOAF
Serves 12-14

Preheat oven to 325 degrees.
Combine in a large bowl:

> 2 pounds ground beef
> 1 pound ground chicken or turkey
> 2 cups finely-torn bread crumbs
> 1/2 cup ketchup
> 1/2 to 3/4 cup water
> 1 egg
> 1 envelope dry onion soup mix
> 1 medium chopped onion
> 1 tsp. salt, if desired

Mix well. Form into two loaves and turn onto a rack on a foil-lined cake pan. Bake for 1 1/2 hours or until a cut through the center shows firm, brown meat.

Variations: Three pounds ground beef may be substituted, or two pounds ground poultry and one pound ground beef, for the meat listed above. Instead of chopped onion, substitute a second envelope of onion soup mix and eliminate salt.

Tips: Bake potatoes, dessert, bread or other hot foods while your meatloaf is cooking to save energy.

OVEN-FRIED POTATOES
Serves 6-8

Preheat oven to 400 degrees.
Peel and dice into small cubes:
6 large baking potatoes

Microwave potatoes until partially cooked.
Place in large bowl. Pour in:
3 Tbsp. oil or melted margarine
1 package onion soup mix

Blend well. Mix in diced meat and/or vegetables of your choice. Place in large metal cake pan. Bake for 30 minutes, stirring occasionally, until mixture is browned and potatoes are tender.

Variations: More or less oil may be used. Serve with or without meat.

Tips: To hurry up the cooking, microwave potatoes until almost done, then broil in the oven, checking carefully to avoid burning.

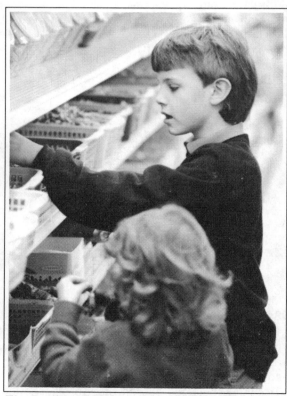

The Barfield children enjoy choosing five pieces of penny candy each, their shopping day treat.

SALMON CROQUETTES
Serves 4-6

Combine in a bowl:
>1 15-ounce can salmon, bones removed
>1 8-ounce can water-packed tuna
>1 egg
>1/4 cup milk
>1 cup crushed saltine crackers

Form mixture into small patties. Crush additional cracker crumbs and roll the patties in extra crumbs. Cover the bottom of a pan with oil to a depth of 1/2 inch. Fry patties in hot oil until golden brown on both sides. Drain thoroughly.

Variations: My mother always deep-fat fried these and they are even more delicious when prepared this way. You can stretch the salmon mixture by changing this recipe as follows: add two slices of shredded bread, a second egg and enough liquid (milk and/or salmon juices) to moisten. Fry as usual.

Tips: If canned salmon is outrageously expensive, try using all tuna, but be prepared for a less tasty entree. To cut down on fat, broil the patties or brown in a nonstick skillet sprayed with cooking spray.

SAUCY GREEN BEANS
Serves 4-6

Fry in a large pan until very crisp:
>4 slices bacon

Saute in bacon grease until tender:
>1 medium chopped onion

Drain grease. Add:
>1/2 cup ketchup
>3 Tbsp. sugar
>Liquid from one can of green beans

Simmer for 15 minutes. Stir in:
>2 15-ounce cans green beans

Simmer an additional 5 to 10 minutes.

Variations: Add more or less bacon as desired.

Tips: This recipe makes a good main dish or side dish, depending on your preference.

STIR-FRY
Serves 6-10

Slice into thin strips:
>4 cups carrots, onions, zucchini, cucumbers, sweet potatoes,
>broccoli,or other fresh produce

In a large frying pan, heat:
>3 Tbsp. oil

When oil is hot enough to sizzle a drop of water, quickly saute vegetables to desired doneness. Stir in:
>2 Tbsp. soy sauce
>2 Tbsp. chunky peanut butter
>1 tsp. garlic powder

Simmer. Combine in an airtight plastic bowl:
>2 Tbsp. cornstarch
>1 cup water

Shake the cornstarch and water together until smooth. Add to vegetables. Bring to a boil, stirring constantly, for one minute. Turn down heat and add cooked leftover meat of your choice. Serve hot over brown rice.

Variations: I like to use this recipe when I'm ready to clean up leftovers, as you can toss in nearly anything on hand. It's not as Oriental with green beans and potatoes, of course, but still tastes good. Most kinds of meat or combination of meats works well, too. One of our favorites is traditional beef/broccoli. Add fresh ginger, if desired.

Tips: To cut down on fat, eliminate the peanut butter and use less vegetable oil.

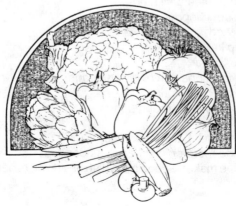

TURKEY BROCCOLI CASSEROLE
Serves 6-8

Preheat oven to 350 degrees. Combine in a saucepan:
> 1 can cream of chicken soup
> 1 cup chicken or turkey broth
> 1 8-ounce package Velveeta cheese

Heat, stirring occasionally, until cheese melts. Set aside. In a separate saucepan, cook until almost tender:
> 1 package frozen broccoli

Set aside. Dice into small pieces:
> 1 to 2 cups leftover turkey

Set aside. In a bowl, prepare:
> 1 package stuffing mix

Place in a greased casserole dish as follows: diced turkey, broccoli, cheese sauce. Top with stuffing. Bake for 20 to 30 minutes, until cheese bubbles and stuffing is lightly browned on top.

Variations and **Tips:** Here's a good example of a recipe that can be altered to save money, with little additional time required. Recently I prepared this dish, and used a basic white sauce (with colby cheese) in place of cream of chicken soup and Velveeta.

Basic White Sauce
Melt in a saucepan:
> 3 Tbsp. reduced calorie margarine

Shake together in an airtight container:
> 1 cup skim milk
> 3 Tbsp. flour
> Dash of salt

Blend into margarine, stirring until bubbly. Add:
> 1 cup sharp cheese, shredded (to make cheese sauce)

Cook and stir just until smooth and thickened.

Instead of packaged stuffing mix, I made my own (see page 92). The broth and turkey pieces came from my freezer, where both were stored when I first cooked the turkey. I also used fresh broccoli.

83

VEGETABLE BEEF SOUP
Serves 6-8

Combine in a Crock-Pot:
>1 pound beef shanks, oxtails, short ribs or beef bones
>1 15-ounce can tomatoes
>2 carrots, sliced
>2 stalks celery, sliced
>2 medium onions, diced
>2 medium potatoes, peeled and diced
>3 cups water
>1 teaspoon salt
>4 whole peppercorns
>3 beef boullion cubes

Cover and cook on low for 12 to 24 hours.

Variations: Use this soup as a catch-all for whatever is in your freezer or refrigerator. The last time I made it, I added leftover ham broth, a little broccoli, a can of green beans, one frozen tomato, and some odds and ends vegetables to the ingredients above. Instead of a Crock-Pot, combine the ingredients in a large kettle, and simmer on the stove all afternoon.

Tips: Serve topped with homemade croutons (see Recipes, page 86).

TUNA SALAD
Serves 4-6

Combine in a bowl:
>1 large can water-packed tuna
>1 hard-boiled egg, diced
>4 Tbsp. mayonnaise
>1 Tbsp. sweet relish
>1 Tbsp. sugar

Chill thoroughly. Serve on oven-toasted buns or French bread.

Variations: Add extra mayonnaise if a creamier texture is desired. Substitute diced chicken or turkey for tuna. Substitute all eggs for meat, and add 1/2 teaspoon paprika. To cut fat, use only egg whites and reduced-fat mayonnaise.

Tips: Serve stuffed in peppers, celery or tomatoes.

BREADS AND BREAKFAST FOODS

BANANA BREAD
Makes 3 thin loaves

Preheat oven to 350 degrees.
Cream together in a large bowl:
>2 cups sugar
>1 cup shortening

Blend in:
>6 ripe bananas, diced
>4 eggs

In a separate bowl, sift together:
>2 1/4 cups flour
>2 tsp. baking soda
>1 tsp. salt

Combine flour mixture with creamed mixture and blend thoroughly. Turn into three greased and floured loaf pans. Bake for 40 to 50 minutes.
Variations: Add nuts and/or raisins.
Tips: To make clean-up easier, I sometimes line the pans with foil and oil with cooking spray. Check for doneness by inserting a toothpick in three or four areas of the bread; if you go through a piece of banana, you may sink into a gooey spot and think the bread isn't done.

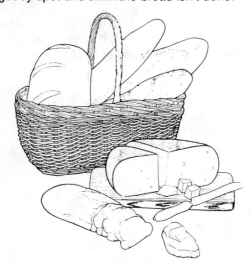

BREADSTICKS/CROUTONS

Breadsticks
Fills a small basket

Preheat oven to 350 degrees. Spread several slices of whole wheat bread on a cookie sheet. Lightly butter one side of each slice. Sprinkle on garlic salt. Cut each slice into five or six narrow rectangles. Bake for about 10 minutes, or until bottom side is browned; turn over and bake another 5 to 10 minutes. Serve hot or cold.

Croutons
Fills a pint jar
Preheat oven to 350 degrees. Dice into small cubes:
> 6 slices thick bread

Place in a large bowl. Add:
> 3 Tbsp. oil
> 1/2 tsp. garlic powder
> Dash of salt

Mix together thoroughly until bread cubes are well coated. Turn onto cookie sheet. Bake for 20 to 30 minutes, stirring occasionally, until crisp.
Variations: Omit or reduce margarine or oil to cut fat. Add other seasonings such as paprika, onion powder, or Parmesan cheese for more flavor.
Tips: Slightly stale bread works a little better than fresh. I keep a plastic bag in the freezer for storing bread ends and leftovers; when the bag is full, I have just enough for a batch of breadsticks or croutons.

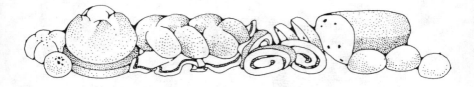

CINNAMON YEAST BREAD (90 MINUTE BREAD)
Makes 4 loaves

Dissolve together in a small, shallow bowl:
>   1 cup very warm water
>   4 packages (or 4 Tbsp.) yeast

Set aside. In a large bowl, combine:
>   3 cups very warm water
>   4 tsp. salt
>   2/3 cup sugar
>   4 Tbsp. oil

Combine the two mixtures. Stir in thoroughly:
>   4 cups whole wheat flour
>   5 cups white flour

Add extra flour a little at a time, just enough to form a soft dough. *Knead by pounding dough vigorously with a large spoon for one minute.* (This is not a mistake!) Form four mounds of dough and let stand. One at a time, roll out each mound with a rolling pin on floured surface to form a rectangle. Sprinkle 3 Tbsp. brown sugar and 1/2 tsp. cinnamon on each rectangle. Start at one of the long ends and roll up tightly to form compact loaves. Tuck loose ends under, seam sides down. Place in four greased bread pans. Let rise, covered in a warm place, for 30 minutes. Bake in preheated 350 degree oven for 30 to 40 minutes.

Variations: This bread can be baked as plain whole wheat bread by eliminating the rolling-out procedure. Simply smooth out the dough and place it directly into pans for rising. All white flour can take the place of half whole wheat, half white flour.

Tips: This is one of my favorite recipes, absolutely delicious! From start to finish takes only 90 minutes or less. It is sometimes difficult to tell when the bread is really done, and you may have to actually cut a loaf in half to make sure there are no doughy areas. Extra loaves freeze well.

CRESCENT ROLLS
Makes 3 dozen rolls

Combine in a small bowl:
>   1/4 cup warm water
>   2 pkg. (or 2 Tbsp.) yeast

Let stand until dissolved. In a separate bowl, combine:
>   3 eggs
>   1 stick melted margarine
>   1 cup milk
>   1/2 cup sugar
>   1 tsp. salt

Combine the two mixtures. Add 4 1/2 cups flour, a little at a time. Mix well. Cover and let rise in a warm, draft-free area until doubled in size. Remove from bowl. Knead until smooth, adding extra flour if required. Divide into three pieces and form into balls. Roll into three circles, one at a time. Spread softened margarine on circle. Slice each circle into 12 pieces as when cutting a pie. Roll up each piece, from wide outer edge to center point, forming crescents. Place crescents on baking sheets. Let rise until doubled. Bake in preheated 350 degree oven for 15 to 20 minutes, until lightly browned.

Variations: Use reduced-fat margarine in place of regular margarine, skim milk in place of whole.

Tips: These tasty rolls should be served and eaten immediately after baking, if possible. For some reason they aren't nearly as good after a day or so. Those I can't use right away I freeze; when reheated, they're almost as delicious as a fresh batch.

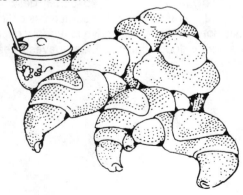

DILL/COTTAGE CHEESE BREAD
Makes 2 loaves

Soften in 1/2 cup warm water:
> 2 packages (or 2 Tbsp.) dry yeast

Set aside. In a separate bowl, combine:
> 4 Tbsp. sugar
> 2 Tbsp. melted margarine
> 1 Tbsp. dry minced onion
> 2 tsp. dill weed
> 2 tsp. salt
> 1/2 tsp. baking soda
> 2 eggs

Combine two mixtures. Heat 2 cups cottage cheese in a saucepan until lukewarm. Add cottage cheese to other ingredients. Slowly add 5 cups flour, a little at a time. Blend well. Cover. Let rise for 50 to 60 minutes in a warm place until doubled in size. Divide dough into two greased loaf pans. Let rise for 30 to 40 minutes. Bake for 30 minutes in a preheated 350 degree oven until golden brown. *Variations:* The original recipe calls for 4 tsp. dill seed in place of 2 tsp. dill weed; I like this milder version better. I sometimes use low-fat cottage cheese. **Tips:** This is a dense, hearty bread and should be baked when the humidity is relatively low for best results.

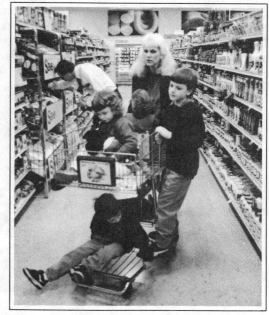

Time for a break on the shopping cart. Well-rested children make a trip to the store more enjoyable.

DONUT MUFFINS
Makes about 3 dozen muffins

Preheat oven to 375 degrees. Cream in a large bowl:
  2 cups sugar
  2/3 cup shortening
  2 eggs
  1 cup milk
Mix together in a separate bowl:
  3 cups flour
  3 tsp. baking powder
  1 tsp. salt
  1/2 tsp. nutmeg

Combine all ingredients and mix thoroughly. Spoon into greased muffin tins, each just over half full. Bake 20 minutes or until tops are lightly browned. While still warm, roll the top of each muffin in melted margarine, then in a mixture of 3/4 cup sugar and 1 tsp. cinnamon.
Variations: I usually substitute cinnamon for nutmeg.
Tips: Donut muffins are so called because they taste much like cake donuts. Fortunately these are much simpler than the genuine homemade version, and much cheaper than store-bought. I use paper baking cups to save time.

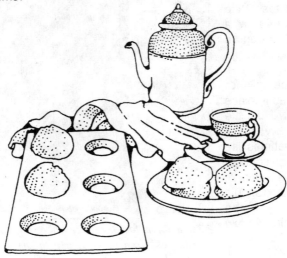

FRENCH BREAD
Makes 4 loaves

In a small bowl, dissolve:
>   2 pkg. (or 2 Tbsp.) dry yeast
>   1 cup very warm water

In a larger bowl, combine:
>   2 cups very warm water
>   2 Tbsp. sugar
>   2 Tbsp. oil
>   3 tsp. salt

Add second mixture to the first and mix well. Stir in 8 cups flour, a little at a time. Work through dough with a large spoon until blended. Add extra flour if needed. Let set for 10 minutes. Stir again thoroughly with spoon. Repeat the stirring process every 10 minutes for three more times, a total of five times in one hour. Turn dough onto floured surface and divide into four pieces. Shape into balls and let rise for 10 minutes. Roll out flat, then roll up firmly. Place on cookie sheets. Score diagonally five times on each top. Let rise until doubled. Bake in a preheated 400 degree oven for 30 to 35 minutes.

Variations: Substitute 2 cups whole wheat flour plus 6 cups white flour, for all white flour.

Tips: Lightly butter the bread tops during the last 10 minutes of baking for a golden crust (I use reduced-calorie margarine).

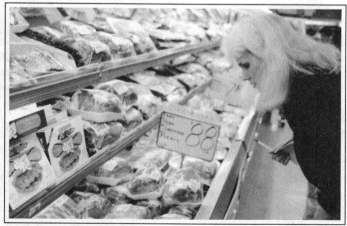

Rhonda tries to follow her own rule, "Always buy meat on sale."

DRY BREAD DRESSING
Serves 8-10

Preheat oven to 350 degrees. Toss together in a large metal cake pan:
>   Several slices of bread, shredded into small pieces
>   1 stick melted margarine
>   1/2 tsp. salt
>   1 to 2 Tbsp. sage, crumbled

Make sure bread pieces are well coated, but not soggy, with margarine and spices. Bake for 30 minutes or until stuffing is dry and a little crunchy. Stir occasionally.

Variations: Reduce or omit the amount of margarine used; I prefer a low-calorie version. Whole wheat bread can be used, as well as leftover buns, rolls and bread ends.

Tips: This is my mother's recipe, and she served it in place of traditional, moister stuffing. I empty my "odds and ends breads" freezer bag when I have enough for a pan's worth of stuffing. If time is short, increase the oven temperature, stir more often and watch closely to avoid burning. Serve with gravy.

GRANOLA
Serves 6-8

Preheat oven to 350 degrees. Combine in a saucepan:
>   3/4 cup brown sugar
>   1/3 cup honey
>   1/3 cup vegetable oil

Heat mixture to boiling. Simmer for about five minutes, stirring occasionally, until oil and sugars blend. In the meantime, combine 5 cups quick oats and 1 tsp. cinnamon. Pour sugar/oil mixture over oats and mix thoroughly. Bake on greased cookie sheets for 20 to 40 minutes, depending on how crispy you like your granola.

Variations: Add nuts, sunflower seeds, coconut, raisins and dried fruit for a wonderful taste. (I omit these things because it drives up the cost considerably.) Add a couple of tablespoons of peanut butter to the sugar/ oil mixture.

Tips: When baking the granola, check often to avoid burning. We have an electric oven and I turn it off after 30 minutes, leaving the granola inside for some time longer. The result is a crunchy delight. I usually double or triple this recipe.

OATMEAL PANCAKES
Serves 4-6

Combine in a large bowl:
> 2 cups flour
> 1/2 cup brown sugar
> 4 tsp. baking powder
> 1/2 tsp. salt

Set aside. In another bowl, beat together:
> 2 eggs
> 1 cup leftover cooked oatmeal
> 2 cups milk
> 1/2 cup oil

Combine the two mixtures and blend until smooth. For each pancake, pour 1/4 cup batter onto greased hot skillet. Cook until bubbles begin to form on top, turn and brown other side.

Variations: This recipe is *very* flexible! Make the batter thicker or thinner, as you prefer. For a treat, add chocolate chips, nuts or bits of banana. Use all or part whole wheat flour instead of all white flour, adding a little extra liquid as needed. Leave out the oil completely if you like; I do sometimes, and substitute more milk instead. You can also omit cooked oatmeal, or replace it with 3/4 cup dry oats soaked in 1/2 cup hot water.

Tips: These pancakes are so moist you don't need syrup. I usually serve them with a dusting of powdered sugar on top. But if you prefer, here's an easy, rich, low-fat recipe.

Pancake Syrup
Combine in a saucepan:
> 3 cups brown sugar
> 1 1/2 cups water
> 1 tsp. vanilla

Bring to a boil and stir constantly until sugar dissolves.

POPOVERS
Makes about 16 popovers

Preheat oven to 450 degrees. Combine in a large bowl:
    1 cup white flour
    1/4 cup sugar
    1/2 tsp. salt
    3 well-beaten eggs
    1 cup milk
    2 Tbsp. melted margarine

Grease muffin tins well and briefly heat in preheated oven. Immediately fill 1/3 full with popover batter. Bake at 450 degrees for 20 minutes, then reduce heat to 350 degrees and bake for an additional 10 to 20 minutes. *Variations:* Margarine may be completely omitted. Popovers can be served as is with jelly or jam, or stuffed with nearly anything imaginable: diced meats, vegetables, cheeses, fruit mixtures, puddings, etc. We enjoy them plain, but these moist, delicious rolls could be the base for a main dish.
Tips: I like this recipe because it's fast, easy and good. Do not open the oven until after 30 minutes of baking or the popovers may fall. It's a little tricky to get them to "puff." It may take you a few tries before you're able to make this work, but even flattened popovers taste wonderful. Do not use paper baking cups!

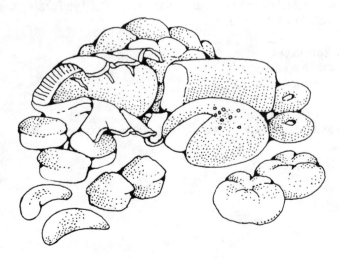

POPPY SEED MUFFINS
Makes about 2 dozen muffins

Preheat oven to 400 degrees. Mix together in a bowl:
>2 cups flour
>3 tsp. poppy seeds
>1/2 tsp. salt
>1/4 tsp. baking soda

In a separate bowl, combine:
>1/2 cup softened margarine
>1 cup sugar
>2 eggs

Cream together thoroughly. Beat in:
>1 cup yogurt
>1 tsp. vanilla

Combine the two mixtures. Spoon into greased muffin tins and bake for 15 to 20 minutes.

Variations: Poppy seeds can be omitted. Use plain yogurt or any flavor you prefer. I have doubled the recipe using only one cup of yogurt (instead of two) by adding a little less flour, with good results.

Tips: Buy your poppy seeds in bulk from a co-op or health food store for a tremendous savings. Homemade yogurt will also save you money (see page 101).

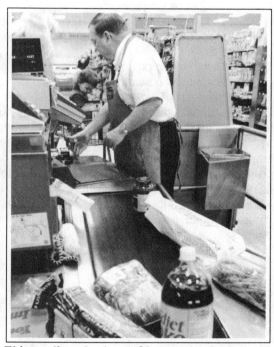

This two-liter of soda cost 35 cents, thanks to a good sale price combined with double coupons. Everthing else pictured was less than half of its regular price.

PUMPKIN / ZUCCHINI BREAD
Makes 2 loaves

Preheat oven to 325 degrees. Grease and flour two loaf pans. Cream together in a large bowl:
> 2 cups sugar
> 1 cup oil

Gradually add:
> 3 eggs
> 2 tsp. vanilla

Beat well. Grate 3 cups pumpkin or zucchini. Add to sugar and oil mixture and blend well.

In a separate bowl, combine:
> 1 1/2 cups white flour
> 1 1/2 cups whole wheat flour
> 1 tsp. cinnamon
> 1 tsp. salt
> 1 tsp. baking powder
> 1 tsp. baking soda

Combine the two mixtures and blend well. Bake for one hour, or until toothpick inserted in the center comes out clean.

Variations: This recipe is an excellent way to use up garden vegetables; I have substituted squash, for example, with good results. Add nuts if you prefer. The amount of oil can be reduced, but the resulting bread is not as moist. All white flour can take the place of half whole wheat, half white.

Tips: My children love this bread and often ask for seconds and thirds. It makes a good, nutritious snack and doesn't take long to make. I usually double the recipe and freeze two of the four loaves.

MISCELLANEOUS RECIPES

FROZEN FRUIT DELIGHT
Serves 8-10

Combine in a blender:
> 2 large, ripe bananas, cut into pieces
> 1 1/2 cups sugar
> 1/2 can orange juice concentrate
> Juice of 2 lemons (or 2 Tbsp. lemon juice)
> 1 small can crushed pineapple
> 3 cups water

Blend until smooth. Pour thin layers into metal trays and freeze. Just before serving, slice into small pieces and thaw slightly.
Variations: Both sugar and lemon juice can be omitted; the resulting frozen fruit is a little more tangy. The original recipe calls for 4 oranges with pulp in place of orange juice. If you have a food processor or the time to prepare the oranges, try this option for additional fiber.
Tips: We often make Frozen Fruit Delight into popsicles.

LEMON GELATIN DELIGHT
Serves 8-10

Combine in a bowl:
> 2 small packages lemon jello
> 4 cups boiling water
> 16 large marshmallows

Stir until dissolved. Cool until thickened. Fold in:
> 1 15-ounce can crushed pineapple, drained (reserve juice)
> 4 thinly sliced bananas

Chill until firm. Make topping by combining in a saucepan:
> 1 cup pineapple juice
> 2 Tbsp. flour
> 2 Tbsp. margarine
> 1/2 cup sugar

Heat slowly, stirring constantly until smooth and thickened. Cool. Add 1 cup whipped topping. Spread entire mixture over gelatin. Chill for an hour or more before serving.
Variations: Any flavor of jello works well. Add leftover fruit or juice you have on hand. Omit the margarine and marshmallows if you like.
Tips: I make this recipe in a large glass cake pan.

JELLO COTTAGE CHEESE SALAD
Serves 8-10

Prepare according to package directions:
　　　1 large box jello, any flavor

Refrigerate until partly set. Stir in:
　　　1 small can crushed pineapple
　　　1 small carton cottage cheese
　　　1 9-ounce container whipped topping

Let set in refrigerator until completely firm.
Variations: Use this recipe as a catch-all for leftover fruits and fruit juices (use juice in place of water called for in the jello recipe). Whipped topping can be completely eliminated.
Tips: Make your own whipped topping if you prefer (below).

Whipped Topping
Makes about 2 cups

Combine in a shallow, chilled bowl:
　　　1 cup cold water
　　　1 tsp. lemon juice
　　　1 package unflavored gelatin
With chilled beaters, gradually blend in:
　　　1 cup nonfat dry milk powder
Whip at high speed until light and fluffy, with soft peaks forming. Gradually add:
　　　1/3 cup sugar
　　　1/2 tsp. vanilla

Serve at once or chill.
Variations: Add a touch of cinnamon or a little more or less lemon juice, as you prefer.
Tips: The taste is good, but I have never been able to make whipped topping with the same consistency as store-bought. Plan to have a more liquid version from this recipe. You may have to beat the whipped topping for several minutes.

MILK SUBSTITUTES AND PRODUCTS

Sweetened Condensed Milk
Mix in a blender until thickened:
> 1 cup dry milk powder
> 1/2 cup boiling water
> 2/3 cup sugar
> 3 Tbsp. melted margarine
> Pinch of salt

Store in a tightly covered container in the refrigerator.

Tips: This recipe yields the same amount as one can of Eagle Brand milk and can be used in any recipe calling for it.

Soured Milk or Buttermilk
Place in an empty one cup container:
> 1 Tbsp. lemon juice
> Fill to the top with milk.

Tips: Use in place of one cup buttermilk or one cup soured milk.

Low-Fat Sour Cream (from *The New Lean Toward Health*)
Combine in a blender:
> 1 cup low-fat cottage cheese
> 1 Tbsp. skim milk
> 2 Tbsp. lemon juice

Blend until smooth.

Tips: Substitute low-fat sour cream for one cup regular sour cream.

SALAD DRESSINGS

Sweet French Salad Dressing
Makes about 3 cups

Combine in a blender:
      1 1/2 cups sugar
      1 1/2 cups vegetable oil
      1/2 cup dark vinegar
      1/2 cup ketchup
      1 tsp. celery seed
      1 tsp. paprika
      1 tsp. salt
      1 tsp. onion juice

Mix together thoroughly.
Variations: Finely-chopped onions can substitute for onion juice. I use 1/2 cup oil and about 1 cup sugar, rather than what's listed in the recipe.
Tips: Store in the refrigerator in a tightly-covered jar. Shake well before serving.

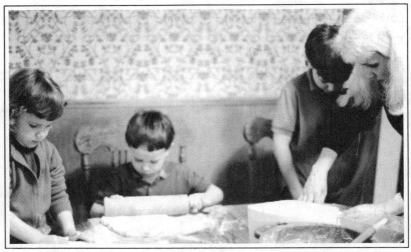

Lisa, Christian and Eric enjoy making bread at a cost of about 35 cents a loaf.

Ranch Salad Dressing
Makes 2 cups

Combine in a blender:
     1 cup mayonnaise
     1 cup buttermilk (see Milk Substitutes recipe)
     2 Tbsp. onion juice
     2 tsp. parsley, finely chopped
     1/4 tsp. salt
     1/4 tsp. garlic powder
     1/4 tsp. paprika
     1/4 tsp. black pepper

Mix well. Store in refrigerator.
Variations: Add more or less spices according to your taste. Substitute low-fat mayonnaise or plain yogurt for regular mayonnaise. I have used 2 Tbsp. onion powder in place of onion juice.
Tips: These two salad dressings are much cheaper than store-bought and delicious!

YOGURT
Makes about 8 cups

Heat in a large saucepan:
     2 quarts milk

Use candy thermometer to gauge when milk reaches 180 degrees. Remove from heat and cool to 112 degrees. Stir in 4 to 6 Tbsp. plain yogurt. Pour into hot, sterilized jars. Meanwhile, preheat oven to 200 degrees, then turn off. Place jars containing yogurt in warm oven. Turn on oven light and leave jars in oven overnight. Yogurt will be ready in the morning.
Variations: Once yogurt is set, blend in any mixture of fruit, syrup or juice you like.
Tips: If you have a yogurt maker, follow the manufacturer's directions and the above recipe. It's best to use whole or 2% milk rather than skim. New yogurt can be made from four to six tablespoons of *your* plain yogurt.

DESSERTS

APPLE CRISP
Serves 8-10

Preheat oven to 375 degrees. Peel and dice:
> 5 pounds apples

Grease a large cake pan. Place apples in pan and sprinkle with:
> 1/2 cup sugar
> 2 tsp. cinnamon

Set aside. In a bowl, combine:
> 1 cup flour
> 1 cup brown sugar
> 1/2 cup rolled oats
> 1/2 cup melted margarine

Mix well, until crumbly. Spoon over apples. Bake for 35 minutes, or until apples are tender and bubbly.

Variations: The amount of margarine used can be reduced. Substitute two cans of apple pie filling for fresh apples and reduce baking time. Use any fruit you like.

Tips: Serve hot or cold, with whipped topping or ice cream. We usually eat ours plain.

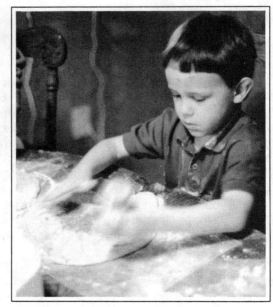

BROWNIES
Serves 8 (small squares)

Preheat oven to 350 degrees. Combine in a bowl:
>3/4 cup margarine, melted
>1 1/2 cup sugar
>1 1/2 tsp. vanilla

Add, one at a time:
>3 eggs

Beat well. In a separate bowl, combine:
>3/4 cup flour
>1/2 cup cocoa
>1/2 tsp. baking powder
>1/2 tsp. salt

Gradually combine two mixtures until well blended. Spread in greased 8 inch pan. Bake for 40 minutes or until brownie begins to pull away from edges of pan. Do not overbake; brownie should look a little gooey.

Variations: Add nuts or marshmallows.

Tips: Sorry, if you're trying to cut back on fat, this is *not* the recipe for you! I like to double the quantities and freeze individual brownies; then when a chocolate craving comes, I have something to satisfy it. These brownies are just as good as the ones at the cookie store, but much cheaper.

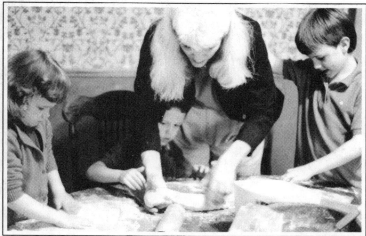

Making cinnamon yeast bread is only a 90 minute project from start to finish (see Recipes, p. 87).

CARAMEL CORN
Fills two large bowls

Preheat oven to 250 degrees. Prepare in a popcorn popper or frying pan:
    6 quarts (2 large bowls) popped corn
Set aside. Combine in a large, heavy-duty saucepan:
    2 cups brown sugar
    2 sticks margarine
    1/2 cup white syrup
    1/4 tsp. cream of tartar
    1/4 tsp. salt

Bring to a rolling boil. Let boil, stirring occasionally, for five minutes. Remove from heat. Add 1 1/2 tsp. baking soda. Mix well. Working fast, stir hot caramel mixture into popped corn until thoroughly blended. Spread on greased cookie sheets. Bake for 30 minutes, stirring once or twice. Remove from oven. When lukewarm, break into small pieces. Cool completely. Store in airtight containers.

Variations: Add peanuts or other nuts. This recipe makes a very rich candy; I like to spread the mixture over 10 to 12 quarts of popcorn (rather than 6) for a lighter variation. If the syrup cools before you are able to spread it all on the popcorn, reheat briefly on the stove.

Tips: This is one of my favorite recipes! Caramel corn can be stored in the freezer for several months or in the refrigerator for a few weeks.

CHOCOLATE CREAMS
Makes four dozen or more

Combine in a medium size bowl:
> 4 cups powdered sugar, sifted
> 1 3-ounce package cream cheese, softened
> 1 stick margarine, softened
> 1 1/2 tsp. vanilla

Beat well with a mixer until creamy and smooth. Form into balls one inch in diameter. Freeze on waxed paper until solid. Then, in the top of a double boiler, melt one 12-ounce package semi-sweet chocolate chips and a one inch square of paraffin. Take a few balls out of the freezer at a time. Place toothpick straight down into the top of each ball, and quickly dip in melted chocolate. Remove toothpick immediately by using a second toothpick as a lever. Cover toothpick hole with a little melted chocolate or a piece of pecan. Add more paraffin to the chocolate mixture as needed to avoid a thick, gummy mixture.

Variations: I have doubled the candy part of the recipe and found 12 ounces of chocolate chips just the right amount to cover all the creams.

Tips: My mother devised this variation of a very complicated fondant recipe. I think they're the best candies I've ever tasted, and are relatively inexpensive and easy to make (though you have to work fast during chocolate dipping). They make delightful holiday presents.

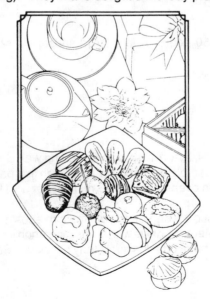

FIVE MINUTE CUSTARD PIE
Serves 6-8

Preheat oven to 350 degrees. Combine in a blender:
    2 cups milk
    4 eggs
    2/3 cup sugar
    1/2 cup flour
    1/3 cup melted margarine
    1/3 cup cocoa
    1 tsp. vanilla
    Pinch of salt
Using part of the margarine and flour, grease and flour two pie pans or ovenproof casserole dishes. Blend mixture a few seconds, until smooth. Pour into pans or dishes. Bake for 30 minutes, or until knife inserted in center comes out clean.
Variations: Omit all but one tablespoon melted margarine. Leave out cocoa and add one cup shredded coconut.
Tips: This recipe actually takes me five minutes to assemble! Best of all, it makes its own crust. Chill for two hours or more before serving.

BAKED CUSTARD
Serves 8-10

Preheat oven to 350 degrees. In a large saucepan, scald until nearly boiling:
5 1/3 cups skim milk
Combine in a large bowl:
1 cup Egg Beaters
1 cup sugar
1/2 tsp. salt

Pour into scalded milk. Add 1 tsp. vanilla. Blend well. Pour custard into large ovenproof casserole dish and place the dish in a pan filled with one inch of water. Set in oven. Bake for 40 minutes, or until knife inserted in center comes out clean.
Variations: One cup's worth of egg whites can substitute for the more expensive Egg Beaters. Sprinkle with a little cinnamon just before baking.
Tips: This low-fat, nutritious dessert is truly delicious. Serve hot or well-chilled, as you like it.

HOT FUDGE PUDDING CAKE
Serves 8-10

Preheat oven to 350 degrees. In a large bowl, sift together:
> 2 cups flour
> 1/3 cup cocoa
> 4 tsp. baking powder
> 1 tsp. salt

Stir in:
> 2 cups sugar
> 1 cup milk
> 1/3 cup oil
> 2 tsp. vanilla

Mix well. Spread into large, greased cake pan. Set aside. In a separate bowl, combine 2 cups brown sugar and 2/3 cup cocoa. Sprinkle topping over cake. Pour 3 cups hot water over all. Bake for 40 to 45 minutes. Finished cake will be gooey! Let set for 10 minutes before serving.

Variations: I cut the amount of cocoa in half in both the cake and the topping, and also reduce the amount of sugar.

Tips: This is definitely a "company dessert," very rich and sweet. Serve with vanilla ice cream or whipped topping.

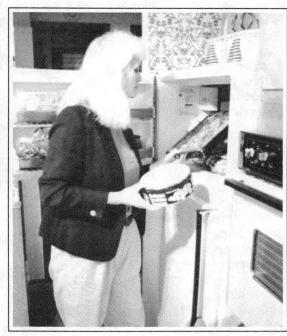

Rhonda takes lasagna and cookies from the stockpile of foods in her freezer.

NO-FAT WHITE CAKE
Serves 8-10

Preheat oven to 350 degrees. Spray a large rectangular cake pan with cooking spray. In a large bowl, combine:
>2 cups flour
>1/2 cup corn starch
>3 tsp. baking powder
>1 tsp. salt

In another bowl, using fork or wire whisk, stir together:
>2 cups sugar
>1 1/3 cups skim milk

When sugar is nearly dissolved, add:
>4 egg whites
>2/3 cup Karo light syrup
>2 tsp. vanilla

Blend thoroughly. Gradually combine mixtures, stirring until smooth. Pour into prepared pan. Bake for 30 minutes or until toothpick inserted in center comes out clean. Cool in pan on wire rack.

Variations: Serve with fresh or frozen fruit and/or whipped topping. It is not necessary to use name brand syrup.

Tips: This cake is light and airy at first, but toughens quickly with age. What you cannot eat immediately, I recommend you freeze. This is one of several delicious dessert recipes printed in *Fat-Free Indulgences*; see Resources.

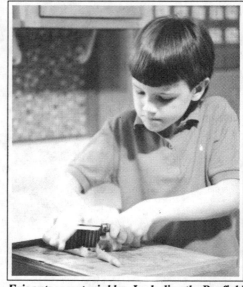

Eric cuts carrot crinkles. Including the Barfield children in cooking has encouraged them to try many new, nutritious foods.

OATMEAL CRISPIES
Makes 4 dozen or more

Preheat oven to 350 degrees. Combine in a large bowl:
>1 cup shortening
>1 cup sugar
>1 cup brown sugar
>2 eggs

Stir in:
>2 cups flour
>2 cups rolled oats
>1 tsp. salt
>1 tsp. baking soda

Mix well. Drop by tablespoonsful onto ungreased cookie sheets. Bake for 8 to 10 minutes, or until very lightly browned.

Variations: Add chocolate chips or raisins to the dough. Use more flour for a puffier kind of cookie; these are thin and crisp. I sometimes use 1/2 cup shortening (rather than one full cup) with no change in taste.

Tips: These cookies freeze very well.

FRUIT COBBLER
Serves 6-8

Preheat oven to 375 degrees. Combine in a bowl:
>1 stick margarine, melted
>1 cup sugar
>1 cup flour
>3/4 cup milk
>1 1/2 tsp. baking powder

Mix well and pour into greased 8" square pan. Top with 1 can pie filling (or 3 cups fresh fruit) and 1 cup sugar. Spoon fruit on top of mixture and do not stir. Bake for 40 to 45 minutes.

Variations: I often use whatever fresh or frozen fruit I have on hand. Both sugar and margarine can be reduced by up to one-third.

Tips: We almost always eat fresh fruit, but this dessert is a nice change. Its taste is similar to that of a fruit pie with much less work.

POUND CAKE
Serves 8-10

Preheat oven to 350 degrees. Have all ingredients at room temperature.
Cream:
>3 sticks margarine

Gradually add:
>2 1/2 cups sugar

Mix thoroughly. Add one at a time:
>5 eggs

Beat continuously until fluffy.
In a separate bowl, combine:
>1 cup milk
>2 tsp. vanilla
>1 tsp. lemon juice

Set aside. In a third bowl, sift:
>3 1/3 cups flour

Add flour alternately with liquids to first mixture. Blend thoroughly. Bake in a tube or Bundt pan for about 50 minutes, or until toothpick in center comes out clean.

Variations: This cake can be baked in any number of different sizes of pans, but remember to reduce cooking time. A little cocoa and extra sugar produce chocolate pound cake.

Tips: The recipe contains no baking powder or soda and so does not rise as much as ordinary cakes. I have found pound cake to be perfect for cut-up birthday and holiday cakes. It slices well and does not crumble, making it easy to assemble pieces and frost the finished product.

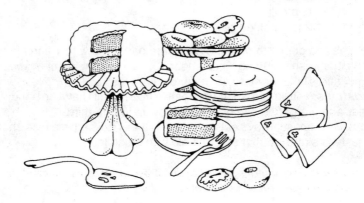

WACKY CAKE
Serves 8-10

Preheat oven to 350 degrees. Sift together in a large bowl:
- 3 cups flour
- 2 cups sugar
- 1/2 cup cocoa
- 2 tsp. baking soda
- 1/2 tsp. salt

Add:
- 2 cups cold water
- 3/4 cup oil
- 2 tsp. vinegar
- 2 tsp. vanilla

Stir with a whisk just until well blended. Pour into large, ungreased cake pan. Bake for 30 to 35 minutes, or until toothpick inserted into center comes out clean.

Variations: I sometimes omit the cocoa and add a second teaspoon of vanilla.

Tips: This is my five minute cake! Since there are no eggs, mixing time is only a few seconds and can even be done with a fork. Wacky cake actually becomes moister the longer it sits. Serve frosted, with whipped topping or plain.

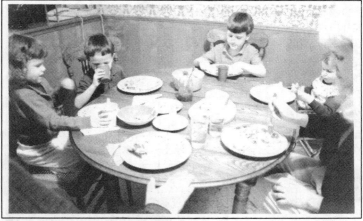

Dinner is served: lasagna, lettuce and broccoli salad, carrot crinkles, cinnamon yeast bread and oatmeal cookies.

PEAK SEASON FOR FRUITS & VEGETABLES

	JANUARY	FEBRUARY	MARCH	APRIL	MAY	JUNE	JULY	AUGUST	SEPTEMBER	OCTOBER	NOVEMBER	DECEMBER
FRUIT												
Apples									■	■	■	■
Apricot						■	■	■				
Avocados			■	■			■	■	■			
Bananas						■	■					
Blackberries							■	■				
Blueberries							■	■				
Cherries						■	■					
Cranberries										■	■	
Grapefruit	■	■	■	■								
Grapes								■	■			
Lemons						■	■					
Melons							■	■				
Nectarines							■	■				■
Oranges	■	■	■				■					■
Peaches							■	■				
Pears								■	■			
Pineapples			■	■	■							
Plums						■	■	■				
Raspberries				■	■	■						
Strawberries				■	■	■						
Tangerines	■											■
Watermelon						■	■					
VEGETABLES												
Artichokes			■	■								
Asparagus				■	■							
Green Beans				■	■		■	■				
Beets						■	■					
Broccoli	■	■								■	■	■
Brussel Sprouts										■	■	■
Cabbage					■							
Carrots	■	■	■	■	■	■	■	■	■	■	■	■
Celery	■	■	■	■	■	■	■	■	■	■	■	■
Corn							■	■				
Cucumber							■	■				
Eggplant								■	■	■		
Lettuce					■	■						
Mushrooms										■	■	■
Onions					■	■						
Green Onions					■	■	■					
Peas				■	■							
Peppers								■	■	■		
Potatoes	■	■	■									
Pumpkins										■	■	
Spinach			■	■	■	■						
Tomatoes							■	■	■			
Winter Squash							■	■	■	■	■	■

7

Final Words

As of this writing, we have lived in our new house for 19 months. We're continuing to budget $50 a week for food, and most of the time, staying within that budget. Some days it seems almost impossible to spend so little. That's when I remind myself of why we limited ourselves in the first place: in order to transfer dollars from grocery bills to higher-priority areas, like housing.

I spent about $57 on food this week. I wasn't well-organized, and simply overshot my goal. Although we make mistakes, Michael and I continue to try and contain the dollar amount we've set for groceries. It seems the children are eating more every day! I've heard legendary stories about teenagers and the amount of food they consume. It isn't going to be easy, sticking to this budget.

On the other hand, I am excited about the information I've been able to share with you in *Eat Well For $50 a Week*. Many of the strategies in Chapters Two and Three are new to me and seem promising. A combination of money-saving techniques and hard work is essential, if any of us are going to keep our grocery bills at half the national average. But I am convinced this task is not impossible.

Again, $50 a week may be an unrealistic figure for some of you. And perhaps not all of the strategies and cost-cutting ideas apply to your situation; they don't all apply to ours. What I have tried to show is that there are many different approaches to saving money on groceries. I am confident that you will be able to discover what works best for you, and adjust your lifestyle accordingly.

A final chapter should point out that these 144 pages are certainly not the final *word*. I hope to hear from many of you who are more expert than I at saving money on food: write and tell me about any good ideas, recipes or techniques you know (and I don't). Perhaps one of these days, another book will follow from all the new information you've shared.

In the meantime, let me leave you with a checklist to encourage you as you tackle the important job of cutting back on your food budget. What could you do, starting today? What could you do next week? Next month? Nobody will be able to — or want to — do everything on the list. But like our hypothetical Price family, implementing one small step at a time will make a major difference in the amount of money you're spending on groceries. When you add up the savings, it is my sincere hope that you will be able to afford some of the dreams in your life.

CHECKLIST FOR SAVINGS

1) Set up a budget for groceries and plan to spend that total amount weekly.

2) Visit several different stores over a period of a few weeks in order to compare prices.

3) Assemble a notebook that lists each store's prices on products you buy regularly.

4) Make a detailed, well-planned weekly list.

5) Clip coupons and combine them with specials at a double coupon store.

6) Watch for good refund offers on foods you buy, then redeem them.

7) Resolve to shop once a week or less when possible.

8) Stick to your list when you shop.

9) Eliminate impulse buying.

10) Buy generic or store brand products whenever possible.

11) Buy in bulk. This may be as simple as stocking up on supermarket specials.

12) Buy produce that is currently in season.

13) Stock up on fresh, seasonal fruits and vegetables at a pick-your-own place.

14) Stock up on candy right after Halloween, Christmas and other holidays.

15) Never pay full price, wherever you shop.

16) Call around to find alternative food sources in your area.

17) Shop at a warehouse store.

18) Shop at a dairy.

19) Shop at a cheese outlet.

20) Shop at a health food store for some items like spices.

21) Shop at a day-old bread store.

22) Shop at a produce stand.

23) Shop at a meat market that offers special values on meat.

24) Shop at a farmers' market.

25) Try to buy everything on special when you shop at the supermarket.

26) Make out monthly menu plans.

27) Eliminate most convenience foods from your meals.

28) Start making some foods, such as salad dressings and croutons, from scratch.

29) Bake your own bread, by hand or with a breadmaker.

30) Prepare some recipes in large quantities so "convenience foods" are ready in the freezer.

31) Do most of your cooking once every two to four weeks.

32) Keep a careful watch of leftovers and use or freeze excess amounts weekly.

33) Change your diet, substituting a balanced variety of foods for meat.

34) Serve smaller portions of expensive foods.

35) Serve larger portions of healthy, filling foods like brown rice, beans and whole-grain breads.

36) Replace non-nutritious foods, like sugary desserts and white bread, with nutritious ones, like custards and whole wheat bread.

37) Substitute less expensive breakfast items, like oatmeal or French toast, for donuts and fancy cereals.

38) Drink water, brewed tea and Kool-aid rather than boxed fruit drinks, coffee and soda.

39) Eat less.

40) Brown bag some of your family's lunches.

41) Start a garden.

42) Consider becoming a member of a garden club or association.

43) Visit your library or university (county) extension service for free information on gardening, as well as a number of other topics.

44) Be on the lookout for gleaning possibilities.

45) Barter for food with friends and neighbors.

46) Call SHARE headquarters to learn if the organization has a branch in your area.

47) Join a bartering exchange (or at least call and find out more).

48) Join a cooperative.

49) Entertain economically.

50) Eat more meals at home.

51) Limit the amount of money spent on meals away from home.

52) Look over a refunding magazine to see if large-scale refunding and couponing appeals to you.

53) Find out if your family is eligible for any government programs.

54) Read other books and newsletters that will help you to save on your grocery bills.

Happy Savings! — Rhonda Barfield, P.O. Box 665, St. Charles, Missouri 63302-0665.

Appendix One

LISTING OF WAREHOUSE MEMBERSHIP CLUBS

Reprinted with permission from chapter 21 of *How to Save Money On Just About Everything* by William Roberts. See Resources for ordering information. Please remember that as of this writing, all information listed below is current, but may have changed since. I have included only those warehouse clubs that carry some food items.

WAREHOUSE MEMBERSHIP CLUBS

Membership warehouses, or wholesale clubs, are cash and carry operations which normally mark up merchandise about 10 percent above cost, compared to 25 percent or more for discount chains and 50 percent and up for other retailers. As a result of their lower prices, they are another extremely fast growing merchandising segment.

Goods sold by these operators usually are shipped directly from the manufacturer to the warehouse, reducing freight costs and cutting out distributors or other middlemen. There are no salesmen — customers serve themselves, goods are paid for in cash or check, and there are no fancy fixtures. All of these factors generate savings which are passed on to the customer. However, to obtain these savings the buyer may have to purchase some items in larger quantities than he would at other retailers.

Annual sales of discount clubs are estimated at $20 billion and growing. At the time this report goes to press, there will probably be more than 400 discount warehouses in operation in the U.S. with more being added constantly.

WHO CAN JOIN THE CLUB

These operations cater primarily to small businesses and "qualified" individuals. To become an individual member, the applicant usually must belong to a particular group such as a credit union, saver's club, investor's club, government employee's group, community association, utility company employee, senior citizen, etc. As you can see, individual qualifications are written so broadly that it would be hard for an individual not to be able to qualify.

The major players in this market are Price Club, Sam's Wholesale, Costco and PACE. Others (at this writing) include BJ's Wholesale Club, Price Savers, The Wholesale Club, and Warehouse Club. Cities in which these clubs presently operate are shown below. New stores are being added at a rapid clip, so if your town isn't shown, you may want to check with the home office of one or more of the discounters (or your local Chamber of Commerce) to find out if one is planned for your area in the near future.

WHO AND WHERE THEY ARE

BJ's Wholesale Club Inc., One Mercer Road, P. O. Box 3000, Natick, MA 01760. Tel. (617) 651-7400. Membership fees: Business $25.00 annual, individual $25.00 annual.

Warehouses: **Connecticut:** Hartford. **Delaware:** New Castle. **Florida:** Hialeah Gardens, Miami, Sunrise. **Illinois:** Calumet City, Hillside, Niles, Rolling Meadows. **Massachusetts:** Chicopee, Medford, Westboro, Weymouth, North Dartmouth. **New Hampshire:** Salem. **New Jersey:** Maple Shade. **New York:** Albany, Buffalo, East Farmingdale, East Rutherford, North Syracuse, Rochester. **Ohio:** Toledo. **Pennsylvania:** Camp Hill, Philadelphia. **Rhode Island:** Johnston. **Virginia:** Virginia Beach.

Merchandise: Deli, bakery, baking supplies, tobacco, fish, meat, paper, household supplies, canned & frozen foods, spices, tea & coffee, dairy, pet food & supplies, grocery items, health & beauty aids, housewares, soft goods, clocks & watches, books, auto supplies, electronics, office supplies, hardware, small appliances, sporting goods, batteries, film & film processing.

COSTCO Wholesale Corporation, 10809 120th Avenue NE, Kirkland, WA 98033. Tel. (206) 828-8100. Membership fees: Business $25.00 annual, individual $30.00 annual.

Warehouses: **Alaska:** Anchorage. **California:** Bakersfield, Canoga Park, City of Industry, Clovis, Danville, Fremont, Fresno, Garden Grove,

Hawthorne, Lancaster, Martinez, Modesto, Richmond, Riverside, San Bernardino, San Bruno, Sand City, San Jose, San Leandro, Santa Clara, Santa Maria, Santa Rosa, Stockton, Vallejo, Van Nuys, Victorville, Visalia. **Florida:** Clearwater, Davie, Fort Lauderdale, Kendall, Lauderhill, Miami, Orlando, Palm Beach Gardens, Palm Harbor, Pompano Beach, South Orlando, Tampa, West Palm Beach. **Hawaii:** Honolulu. **Idaho:** Boise. **Massachusetts:** Danvers, West Springfield. **Nevada:** Las Vegas, Reno. **Oregon:** Aloha, Clackamas, Eugene, Portland, Tulatin. **Utah:** Salt Lake City. **Washington:** Federal Way, Kenneywick, Kirkland, Lynwood, Seattle, Silverdale, Spokane, Tacoma, Tuykwila, Union Gap. **CANADA:** **Alberta:** Calgary, Edmonton. **British Columbia:** Burnaby, Richmond, Surrey. **Ontario:** Winnepeg.

Merchandise. Apparel, audio & video tapes, beer & wine, books, calculators, cameras, candy, cigarettes, computer supplies, deli products, domestics, drug store items, frozen foods, furniture, giftware, groceries, hardware, housewares, janitorial supplies, jewelry & watches, appliances, meat products, office equipment & supplies, perishables, photo processing, sporting goods, stereos, sundries, supermarket items, televisions, tires & automotive, tools, toys, typewriters.

Pace Membership Warehouse, 3350 Peoria Street, Aurora, CO 80010. Tel. (303) 364-0700. Memberships: Business $25.00 annual, individual $25.00 annual.

Warehouses: **California:** Cathedral City, Chino, Downey, El Monte, Fountain Valley, Fullerton, Gardena, San Bernardino, San Fernando, Woodland Hills. **Colorado:** Arvada, Aurora, Colorado Springs, Fort Collins, Sheridan. **Connecticut:** Berlin. **Florida:** Hillsborough County, Palm Harbor, Pinellas Park, Tampa. **Georgia:** Forest Park, Marietta, Norcross, Roswell, Stone Mountain. **Iowa:** Des Moines. **Kentucky:** Lexington, Louisville. **Maryland:** Baltimore (2), Capitol Heights, Landover, Laurel. **Michigan:** Farmington Hills, Flint, Kalamazoo, Madison Heights, Roseville, Saginaw, Taylor, Westland, Ypsilanti. **Nebraska:** Omaha. **New York:** Cheektowaga. **North Carolina:** Cary, Charlotte (2), Greensboro. **Ohio:** Cincinnati, Cleveland (2), Toledo. **Pennsylvania:** Hatboro, Langhorne, Monroeville, Ross Township, West Miffin. **Rhode Island:** Warwick.

Merchandise: Office equipment & supplies, fresh produce, furniture, tires & auto supplies, TVs, VCRs, stereos, jewelry & watches, clothing, linens, groceries & frozen foods, tobacco products, sundries, hardware, housewares, janitorial supplies, appliances, health & beauty aids, sporting goods, toys, books.

Price Club, 2647 Arianne, San Diego, CA 92117. Tel. (619) 581-4600. Memberships: Business $25.00 annual, individual $25.00 annual.

Warehouses: **Arizona:** Glendale, Mesa, Phoenix, Scottsdale, Tempe, Tucson (2). **California:** Alhambra, Azusa, Bakersfield, Burbank, Chula Vista, Coachella Marcos, Santee, Signal Hill, South San Francisco, Sunnyvale. **Colorado:** Aurora, Westminster. **Connecticut:** North Haven. **Maryland:** Gaithersburg, Glen Burnie, Baltimore, Beltsville, Suitland. **New Jersey:** Edison, Mapleshade. **New Mexico:** Albuquerque. **New York:** Cheektowaga, Copiague, Smithtown. **Virginia:** Fairfax, Hampton, Loudoun, Norfolk, Richmond, South Richmond.

Merchandise: Office equipment & supplies, restaurant supplies, computer supplies, typewriters, calculators, tools, janitorial supplies, food, frozen food, perishables, wine, spirits, sundries, books, jewelry, appliances, housewares, giftware, clothing, automotive supplies, tires, sporting goods.

Price Savers Wholesale Warehouse, 986 Atherton Drive, Suite 220, Salt Lake City, UT 84123. Tel. 1-801-466-7777. Memberships: Company $25.00 annual; individual—no fee but prices are 5% higher than member's unless individual buys a PlusCard for a $30.00 annual fee.

Warehouses: **Alaska:** Anchorage. **Arizona:** Gilbert, Phoenix (3). **California:** City of Industry, Irvine, Montclair, Rancho Cordova, Sacramento, South Gate, Stanton. **Utah:** Murray, Ogden, Provo, Salt Lake City. **Washington:** Fife, Seattle.

Merchandise: Frozen foods, deli, dairy products, bakery items, snacks, produce, spirits, condiments, office supplies & furniture, computers, typewriters, calculators, entertainment centers, lamps, paper, cleaning supplies, vacuums, household supplies, electronics, appliances, hardware, tools, health & sports equipment, and automotive supplies.

Sam's Wholesale Club, c/o Wal-Mart Stores Inc., Bentonville, AR 72712. Tel. (501) 273-4000. Membership: Company $25.00 annual.

Warehouses: **Alabama:** Birmingham, Huntsville, Irondale, Mobile, Montgomery. **Arkansas:** Little Rock, Fort Smith, North Little Rock, Springdale. **Colorado:** Colorado Springs, Loveland. **Florida:** Daytona Beach, Fern Park, Fort Myers, Fort Pierce, Gainesville, Jacksonville (2), Lakeland, Lantana, Melbourne, Orlando, Panama City, Pensacola, Sarasota, Tallahassee. **Georgia:** Atlanta, Augusta, Austell, Columbus, Duluth, Macon, Marietta, Savannah. **Illinois:** Joliet, Naperville, Peoria, Streamwood, Matteson, Springfield, O'Fallon, Rockford. **Indiana:** Evansville, Fishers, Goshen, Lafayette, Merrillville, Terre Haute. **Iowa:** Cedar Rapids, Davenport. **Kansas:** Lenexa, Wichita. **Kentucky:** Florence, Jeffersontown, Louisville. **Louisiana:** Baton Rouge, Harvey, Kenner, Lake Charles, Monroe, New Orleans, Scott, Shreveport (2). **Michigan:** Flint, Lansing. **Mississippi:** Gulfport, Jackson. **Missouri:** Columbia, Ferguson, Grandview, Kansas City (2), Springfield, St. Charles, St. Louis. **Nebraska:** Omaha. **New Jersey:** Atlantic City, Delran Township. **North Carolina:** Fayetteville, Matthews, Raleigh, Wilmington, Winston-Salem. **North Dakota:** Fargo. **Ohio:** Cincinnati (2), Dayton, Holland. **Oklahoma:** Lawton, Midwest City, Oklahoma City (2), Tulsa. **Pennsylvania:** Temple, York. **South Carolina:** Columbia, Greenville, North Charleston, Spartanburg. **South Dakota:** Sioux Falls. **Tennessee:** Chattanooga, Kingsport, Knoxville, Memphis (2), Nashville (2). **Texas:** Abilene, Amarillo, Austin (2), Beaumont, Brownsville, Corpus Christi, Dallas (3), El Paso (2), Fort Worth, Grand Prairie, Houston (5), Laredo, Lubbock, Meadows, Midland, Pharr, Plano, Richland Hills, San Antonio (3), Texarkana, Tyler, Waco, White Settlement, Wichita Falls. **Virginia:** Roanoke. **West Virginia:** Cross Lanes. **Wisconsin:** Brookfield, Franklin, Green Bay, Madison.

Merchandise: Office supplies, computer equipment, food products, frozen foods, tires & batteries, auto supplies, televisions, camcorders, VCRs, major appliances, small appliances, home furnishings, designer clothing, sheets & towels, small building equipment, hardware, candy, snack items, watches & jewelry.

Warehouse Club, 7235 N. Linder Avenue, Skokie, IL 60077. Tel. (708) 679-6800. Memberships: Business $25.00 annual, individual $35.00, or individuals may elect to pay 5% higher prices instead of membership fee.

Warehouses: **Illinois:** Bridgeview, Niles. **Indiana:** Hammond. **Michigan:** Allen Park, Hazel Park, Redford Township. **Ohio:** Akron, Columbus (2), Dayton. **Pennsylvania:** Bridgeville, North Versailles.

Merchandise: Apparel, linens, office supplies, furniture, appliances, tools, automotive supplies, electronics, video and audio tapes, snack foods, health & beauty aids, tobacco, alcoholic beverages, soft drinks, household supplies, groceries, seasonal items.

The Wholesale Club, 7260 Shadeland Station, Indianapolis, IN 46256. Tel. (317) 842-0351 or (317) 842-0351, ext. 111 for membership information. Membership: Business $25.00 annual.

Warehouses: **Indiana:** Carmel, Fort Wayne, Greenwood, Indianapolis (2), South Bend/Mishawaka. **Michigan:** Kentwood, Portage. **Minnesota:** Burnsville, Fridley, Hermantown, Inver Grove Heights, St. Louis Park, White Bear Lake. **Ohio:** Bedford, Boardman, Brook Park, Columbus (2), Eastlake, Elyria/Lorain, Niles, North Canton. **Wisconsin:** Grand Chute, Menomonee Falls, West Allis.

Merchandise: Apparel, beverages, books, calculators, cheese & dairy, film, frozen foods, hardware & tools, health & beauty aids, home furnishings, housewares, institutional foods, janitorial supplies, jewelry, luggage, major appliances, microwaves, office furniture & supplies, photo processing, sporting goods, stereo & CD players.

Appendix Two

MORE REAL-LIFE SHOPPING LISTS AND MENU PLANS

One week's shopping list and menu plans are described in Chapter One. For those of you who want to learn more about how I shop and cook, here are three additional weeks of actual lists and menus.

SHOPPING LIST #2

From Aldi

3 gallons 2% milk	1 8-ounce package mozzarella cheese
2 pounds stick margarine	1 small container strawberry yogurt
1 box graham crackers	1 box saltine crackers
1 package cheese puffs	1 package tortilla chips
1 package corn chips	1 jar peanut butter
1 bag popcorn	2 pounds brown sugar
5 pounds flour	1 can chicken noodle soup
1 box raisins	1 8-pack hamburger buns
3 loaves whole wheat bread	1 box crisp rice cereal
1 box puffed wheat cereal	1 can frozen orange juice

Total: $23.94

From National

1 pound ground chicken	3 pounds ground beef
3 packages deli turkey	1 medium container low-fat cottage cheese
2 dozen eggs	1 pound baking cocoa
1 small pkg. artificial sweetener	1 package paper baking cups
3 8-ounce cans tomato sauce	1 envelope spaghetti seasoning mix
3 cans name brand vegetables	6 ears sweet corn
1 small loaf day-old herb bread	1 small bag day-old donuts

Total: $19.83

From Sunnyside Produce

2 large bunches bananas   1 large bunch fresh broccoli

Grand Total: $46.02

This week I shopped at Aldi as usual. Their private label cheese, packaged in eight-ounce bags, is actually cheaper per ounce than most co-ops' bulk buy cheese. I can't say that it tastes better, but it does cost less. The same is true of Aldi's tortilla chips in 12-ounce bags; they're cheaper than Sam's Club's version. This was one of the surprising discoveries I made when first comparing prices.

My second stop was a regular supermarket a mile down the road. National's everyday prices tend to be among the highest in town, but the store has some outstanding sales, day-old bread and a bin of meat that's marked down significantly. Because of these factors and a convenient location, I shop there regularly. At National, I bought sweetener, ground beef, cocoa and paper baking cups at regular prices. Everything else was on sale at a 30 to 50% savings. The deli turkey meat was marked down 75% off normal cost. I was able to purchase three cans of tomato sauce and spaghetti seasoning mix for about half of Prego's cost, and decided to give "homemade" a try.

Our refrigerator was still well stocked with a variety of fresh fruit from the week before. On my way home I made a three minute stop at a favorite produce stand and picked up two other items I needed. As I mentioned earlier, I make it a point not to travel far out of my way.

If you're matching up my shopping lists with the corresponding menu plans, you may find a few discrepancies. Some of what I buy is set aside especially for my husband. Michael works well into the wee hours of the morning and has "dinner" when he comes home. There are extra groceries stocked in the cupboard or leftovers waiting on plates for our hungry breadwinner.

WEEKLY MENU #2

July 22

  B: Cold cereal with milk
  S: Pancakes from McDonalds
  L: Turkey sandwiches, cheese puffs, bananas, milk
  S: Watermelon slices

D: Hashbrowns (with zucchini, onions and a bit of ground beef added)*, peas, homemade French bread*, zucchini bread*, no-fat white cake*

July 23

B: Oatmeal and granola*, raisins, milk
S: Crackers (at a friend's house)
L: Nachos and cheese, pretzels, canned pears, milk
S: Orange juice popsicles
D: Spaghetti and meat sauce*, lettuce wedges with salad dressing*, zucchini bread*, oatmeal crispies*

July 24

B: Scrambled eggs, toast, milk
S: Apples
L: Turkey roll-ups, crackers, orange slices, milk
S: Oatmeal crispies*
D: Hamburgers and hot dogs, oven-fried potatoes*, carrots, green beans, oatmeal crispies*

July 25

B: Crepes, milk
S: Watermelon slices
L: Peanut butter and jelly sandwiches, potato chips, applesauce, milk
S: Graham crackers
D: Takeout pizza, lemon gelatin salad*, yellow cake

July 26

B: Cold cereal with milk
S: Orange juice
L: Grilled cheese sandwiches, cheese puffs, pickles, milk
S: None
D: Meatloaf*, corn on the cob, breadsticks*, poppy seed muffins*, yellow cake and ice cream

---

* Starred items can be found in Recipes. Check the Recipe Index for an exact page number.

July 27

- B: Oatmeal and granola*, milk
- S: Bananas
- L: Cheese and crackers, raisins, lemon gelatin salad*, milk
- S: Orange juice popsicles
- D: Lasagna*, toasted bagels, lettuce with salad dressing*, candy

July 28

- B: English muffins, scrambled eggs, milk
- S: Watermelon slices
- L: Leftover lasagna*, peanut butter and jelly sandwiches, pretzels, oranges, milk
- S: Grapes and bananas
- D: Salmon croquettes*, broccoli, corn muffins, sugar cookies (from the freezer)

This week's menus require some explanation. A friend of mine, proofreading our daily fare, was horrified at all the beef we ate. I confess! I should have served more chicken and fish and maybe a meatless meal! But it isn't as terrible as it may first appear. Our spaghetti, for example, contained about a half pound ground beef total for all six of us. Even our meatloaf was one-third ground turkey.

I used quite a bit of the deli turkey for sandwiches for the adults. Michael and I tend to eat most of the leftovers, while the children have more variety.

Eric, Christian, Lisa and I took advantage of low-cost food at the restaurant next door, in a second night out for 25 cent hot dogs and burgers. It was blistering hot and this gave me a perfect excuse not to warm up the kitchen, cooking. The pancakes from McDonalds were free, a prize earned by the children through a generous summer reading program at our library. The pizza cost us less than $12 for two large takeouts, Kool-aid and breadsticks.

We splurged on ice cream from the convenience store down the hill. Add another $2.69 to our weekly bill.

Our neighbor Eve very generously shared some produce that was given to her. I added diced zucchini and onions to hash browns, spaghetti sauce and meatloaf. I find that we don't miss some of the meat in a recipe when it's loaded with chunky vegetables. We also dined on zucchini bread, and Michael ate several garden-grown tomatoes as snacks. I sliced cucumbers and placed them in commercial pickle juice (left over from our last two jars of store-bought pickles) with good results.

SHOPPING LIST #3

From Aldi

3 gallons 2% milk

1 12-ounce package colby cheese

2 pounds stick margarine

1 box animal crackers

1 package tortilla chips

1 package potato chips

1 box muffin mix

1 8-pack hamburger buns

1 bottle vegetable oil

5 pounds flour

1 package marshmallows

1 large container oats

3 cans green beans

1 head lettuce

2 dozen eggs

1 container sour cream

1 container raspberry yogurt

1 box saltine crackers

1 package pretzels

1 package corn chips

4 loaves whole wheat bread

1 bottle pure vanilla

1 large bottle ketchup

5 pounds sugar

2 packages dry onion soup mix

3 boxes cold cereal

1 can orange juice concentrate

Total: $28.24

From National

2 pounds ground beef

1 small bottle Karo syrup

6 pack day old bagels

1 large box artificial sweetener

Whole watermelon

2 pounds round steak, half-price

Total: $11.97

From C. Rallo Meat Company

2 1/2 pounds chuck roast

1 pound bacon

Total: $5.20

From Sunnyside Produce

1 head broccoli	4 large apples
3 potatoes	4 ears sweet corn
1 large bunch bananas	
Small bunch grapes	

Total: $3.50
Grand Total: $48.91

This was a four-store week! Fortunately, Aldi and the meat market are only a few yards apart, National a mile down the street, and the produce stand right on my way home. Shopping lasted a little less than two hours.

I've explained more in Chapter Five about my philosophy of taking children along to the grocery store. For the most part mine are well-behaved, so much so that older ladies sometimes compliment our good manners. And then there are bad days, like the time Lisa, age two, threw a full-blown tantrum. Or recently, when an incompetent clerk took 20 minutes to check us out. It wouldn't have been so bad if Mary wasn't fussing and squirming in my arms while I tried to keep her out of the candy bars! In spite of some bad experiences, though, we usually enjoy ourselves in stores.

National had reduced prices on bagels and round steak. I also got a bargain on the watermelon, and the produce manager even cut it in half to make sure ours was a good one. The meat market ran specials on chuck roast and bacon; they were about 40% cheaper than usual, and too good to pass up. (I still had plenty of turkey, chicken and fish in the freezer.) I bought fruit in season at the produce stand for a very low price.

WEEKLY MENU #3

July 29

- B: Cold cereal with milk
- S: Bananas
- L: Leftover meatloaf*, animal crackers, yogurt*, milk
- S: Carrot sticks
- D: Takeout pizza, pound cake* and ice cream

July 30

B: Oatmeal and granola*, raisins, milk
S: Graham crackers
L: Tortilla chips with melted cheese, applesauce, milk
S: Orange juice popsicles
D: Enchiladas* with diced vegetables and beans, shredded lettuce, zucchini sticks, cheese, dip, pound cake* and ice cream

July 31

B: Scrambled eggs, English muffins, toast, milk
S: Watermelon slices
L: Peanut butter and jelly sandwiches, pretzels, milk
S: Grapes
D: Fish sticks, corn on the cob, toasted bagels, oatmeal crispies* (from the freezer)

August 1

B: Oatmeal pancakes*, milk
S: Crisp rice cereal bars
L: Grilled cheese sandwiches, potato chips, milk
S: Orange juice popsicles
D: Dinner out at Taco Bell

August 2

B: Cold cereal with milk
S: Watermelon slices
L: Turkey squares, cheese squares, crackers (make your own "sandwich" ingredients), raisins, milk
S: Bananas
D: Pork in barbeque sauce* on toasted buns, tomato slices, green beans, chocolate cookies

August 3

B: Oatmeal, granola*, raisins, milk
S: Apple slices
L: Chicken noodle soup, crackers, pears, milk

S: Orange juice

D: Tuna salad*, breadsticks*, vegetables (cucumbers, carrots, zucchini) with dip, chocolate cookies

August 4

B: Scrambled eggs, toast, milk

S: Animal crackers

L: Peanut butter and jelly sandwiches, tortilla chips, milk

S: Orange juice popsicles

D: Chicken and noodles, broccoli, five minute custard pie*

Menus this week reflect some special occasions: a birthday on the 29th, and another the following day. We enjoyed restaurant food twice in one week, very unusual for us, but a treat afforded by money gifts. We bought our ice cream on sale at the convenience store down the hill (an extra $2.69).

Some of you may wonder if I spend all my time in the kitchen. Actually, cooking is rather low on my priority list compared to homeschooling and working at my business. To save time, I utilize fast, easy recipes and bake in large quantities. On Lisa's birthday in early July, for example, I made a double recipe of pound cake and froze a sheet cake for Eric's birthday on the 29th. Most of the time I can go to the freezer and pull out something last-minute, if needed, for dinner. This is part of my plan to eliminate store-bought convenience foods. I make my own.

I also clean as I cook. For my own sanity I use paper baking cups, nonstick pans and copper mesh scrubbers. I find myself much more enthusiastic about being in the kitchen if I don't have to face an enormous mess afterward.

SHOPPING LIST #4

From Aldi

4 gallons 2% milk

2 pounds stick margarine

1 large carton cottage cheese

1 package corn chips

1 package pretzels

2 dozen eggs

1 carton blueberry yogurt

1 12-ounce package colby cheese

1 package potato chips

1 package nacho chips

1 box animal crackers	1 box graham crackers
1 bag marshmallows	1 small box jello
2 pounds brown sugar	2 pounds powdered sugar
5 pounds granulated sugar	1 can cream of mushroom soup
1 package corn muffin mix	3 loaves whole wheat bread
2 packages sliced turkey meat	1 large jar applesauce
1 can pineapple	1 can frozen orange juice conc.
1 large container oats	4 boxes cold cereal
1 head lettuce	2 pounds carrots

Total: $36.38

From IGA

1 package jumbo hot dogs	7 pounds ground beef
1 container baking cocoa	1 loaf day-old French bread
1 package day-old dinner rolls	

Total: $11.63

From Sunnyside Produce

1 bunch broccoli	6 small oranges
7 pounds bananas	3 pounds grapes

Total: $3.67
Grand Total: $51.68

Yes, it is the undeniable truth: I went $1.68 over budget this week. With paper products included, I was actually at about $57.00. Sometimes, when we have a little extra money on hand, I spend it! Then again, sometimes I total *less* than $45, so my average is below $50 for food expenditures. And I do have a pretty good excuse, I think: we entertained two guests on both August 9th and 11th for dinner. (Maybe I should have taken my own advice from Chapter Five, "I Can't Save Money on Groceries Because...!")

This week I bought the usual staples at Aldi. IGA had a 99 cents per pound sale on ground beef, so I stocked up. I formed about half the package into patties made with diced onions and flour, freezing some. We grilled a large number of hamburgers and also froze some cooked portions. The rest of the meat I fried with diced onions and other leftover vegetables on hand, drained the grease, and froze in Ziploc bags. From seven pounds of ground beef I was able to make at least five meals — or main parts of meals — for future use. Here again is my "convenience food" that's ready to use in enchiladas, spaghetti or any other number of quick recipes.

IGA turkey hot dogs were on sale, as were the two packages of bread and rolls. At the produce stand I bought three big bunches of bananas at five pounds for $1.00. Some I made into a triple batch of Frozen Fruit Delight (see Recipes), and the rest we ate as snacks.

WEEKLY MENU #4

August 5
- B: Cold cereal with milk
- S: Animal crackers
- L: McDonalds Happy Meal, bananas, milk
- S: Watermelon slices
- D: Grilled hamburgers and hot dogs, relish tray (tomatoes, lettuce, cucumbers, onions), potato chips & dip, baked beans, strawberries

August 6
- B: Oatmeal, granola*, raisins, milk
- S: Bananas
- L: Nachos and melted cheese, applesauce, milk
- S: Orange juice popsicles
- D: Leftover beans and rice, cinnamon yeast bread*, green beans, hot fudge pudding cake*

August 7
- B: Waffles, milk
- S: Bananas
- L: Leftovers, cinnamon yeast bread*, milk
- S: Orange juice and popcorn
- D: Stir-fry* with beef/broccoli, rice, dinner rolls, hot fudge pudding cake*

August 8
- B: Oatmeal pancakes*, milk

S: Watermelon slices
L: Tuna salad* sandwiches, cheese squares, crackers, pretzels, milk
S: Orange juice
D: Leftover hamburgers, cucumbers, corn, jello cottage cheese
salad*, yellow cake

August 9

B: Cold cereal with milk
S: Special dry cereal (a gift from a friend)
L: Fritos with melted cheese, raisins and (dry) cereal, milk
S: Orange juice popsicles
D: Chicken in barbeque sauce*, oven-fried potatoes*, lettuce salad,
cinnamon yeast bread* (from the freezer), praline crunch on ice
cream

August 10

B: Oatmeal and granola*, raisins, milk
S: Popcorn
L: Peanut butter and jelly sandwiches, cheese puffs, grapes, milk
S: Frozen fruit* popsicles
D: Dinner out

August 11

B: Cold cereal with milk
S: Frozen fruit* in cones
L: Grilled cheese sandwiches, cheese puffs, grapes and bananas, milk
S: Animal crackers
D: Roast beef, potatoes, carrots and onions, gravy*, dill/cottage
cheese bread*, fried summer squash, chocolate cookies (from
the freezer)

On August 5th we enjoyed a free McDonalds meal, another summer
reading program prize that we split between the children. Baby Mary
wasn't too interested in the hamburger or soda, though she did wolf down
a couple of french fries. Strawberries from my freezer were a gift from
friends who raided a pick-your-own farm at the very end of the season,

when fruit was free.

I took inventory and decided our jam-packed refrigerator needed a reprieve. My rule is to use it, freeze it or give it away (maybe to the birds or buried in the garden, but that's as a last resort). We ate some form of leftovers for four meals. Produce from our neighbor was either consumed or frozen. At last we could see the shelves again.

As a family, we make a real effort not to waste any food, be it in the refrigerator or at the table. Michael and I take small enough portions to ensure we finish what we have. For the children, teaspoonsful are more in order, at least until we see how much they eat. What is the point of piling on mounds of vegetables, only to have them dumped in the garbage? We have a firm rule that no child receives dessert unless he eats all his vegetables. He doesn't have to eat anything else, and if he is obviously not hungry but *does* eat vegetables, we give him a very small dessert! This strategy is practical, it works and it avoids food fights at the table.

These shopping lists and menu plans were recorded, as I write now, nearly nine months ago. Since then I believe our meals have improved. I have substituted more chicken, turkey, fish and bean dishes in place of ground beef, and I can't remember the last time I bought hot dogs. We eat more whole grain breads and less "chips and dip" than we did last summer. I have also made an effort to increase our servings of fruits and vegetables to five — rather than four — a day, as the American Cancer Society recommends. What about desserts? Well, we've converted to more low-fat puddings, custard pies and similar dishes, but we have a way to go. Nobody's perfect!

Resources

Books, Booklets, Brochures

All About Vegetables

Ortho's comprehensive publication (whose name is self-explanatory) is available in retail stores nationwide, including K-Mart, Builders Square and many others.

Baker's Easy Cut-Up Party Cakes

This full-color, 95 page booklet shows you how to make simple, professional-looking cakes from scratch. You'll save more than the booklet's cost when you make your first cake! Send $2.50 plus your name and address (zip required) to Kraft General Foods USA, P.O. Box 4114, Kankakee, IL 60902.

The Best of The Cheapskate Monthly, Simple Tips For Living Lean in the '90s

Mary Hunt, editor of *Cheapskate Monthly* newsletter, details a 200 page plan for turning your finances around. Features include a step-by-step program for getting out of debt and staying there, plus information on subjects as diverse as coupons, discount shopping, insurance policies and more. The book is available in all bookstores and wherever paperback books are sold.

Cheap Eating

Pat Edwards describes her book as a way to "feed your family well and spend less." *Cheap Eating* goes into more detail than *Eat Well* on growing and preserving your own food. There are also several excellent low-cost recipes. Call Upper Access Books, 1-800-356-9315, for ordering information.

DC Super Heroes Super Healthy Cookbook

Mark Saltzman, Judy Garlan and Michele Grodner have compiled a 100 page classic cookbook of "good food kids can make themselves." Full-color photographs, easy instructions and super hero cartoons on nearly every page inspire young cooks to head for the kitchen. This book is no longer in print, but your local library may either have a copy on hand or locate one through interlibrary loan.

Dinner's in the Freezer!

256 pages in an 8 1/2 x 11 inch format, *Dinner's in the Freezer!* picks up where *Once-a-Month Cooking* leaves off. Jill Bond, author, shares her expertise as a mega-cook who sometimes prepares up to six months' worth of economical, nutritious meals. The book emphasizes a strong Christian world view. Send an SASE for more information. If you prefer to order *Dinner's In The Freezer!*, mail $18.00 plus $2.00 (fourth-class postage) to The Bonding Place, PO Box 736, Lake Hamilton, FL 33851. Or ask for a free sample copy of the Bonds' newsletter by mailing them your name, address and signature.

Extending the Table...A World Community Cookbook

Written in the same format as *More-with-Less Cookbook*, Joetta Handrich Schlabach presents recipes from countries around the world, most of them low-cost. Order her collection through your local Christian bookstore.

Fat-Free Indulgences

For a free brochure with seven delicious fat-free dessert recipes from Karo Corn Syrup, write to *Fat-Free Indulgences*, Dept. K-FFP, P.O. Box 307, Coventry, CT 06238.

The Frugal Mind

This 320 page book by Dr. Charlotte Gorman, subtitled "1,479 Money Saving Tips for Surviving the 1990s," sells for $16.95 + $2.95 shipping and handling (Texas residents add $1.39 sales tax). Send your check or money order to Nottingham Books, Department IBOB, P.O. Box 2454, Denton, TX 76202.

Gardening By Mail

Houghton Mifflin's detailed sourcebook lists all sorts of gardening supplies available through mail-order. Check your local libary's reference department.

How To Save Money on Just About Everything

William Roberts' 208 page book sells for $12.95 + $2.00 shipping and handling (California residents add $1.00 for sales tax). Appendix One in this book is a reprint of most of his chapter 21, "Warehouse Membership Clubs." Send a check or money order to Strebor Publications, P.O. Box 475, Laguna Beach, CA 92652.

More-with-Less Cookbook

Doris Janzen Longacre's cookbook is subtitled "suggestions by Mennonites on how to eat better and consume less of the world's limited food resources." Over 300 pages of recipes and information, the book costs $14.95. It is available from most Christian bookstores, or call 1-800-759-4447.

The New Lean Toward Health

This informative booklet is available from Project LEAN (Low-Fat Eating For America Now, sponsored by the National Center for Nutrition and Dietetics of The American Dietetic Association). Subtitled "Quick, Easy, and Delicious Ways To Reduce the Fat in Your Diet," *The New Lean Toward Health* "gives some practical tips to help make low-fat eating an everyday habit...things to do when shopping for food, cooking, and eating out." See National Center for Nutrition and Dietetics for ordering information.

Once-a-Month Cooking

Written by Mimi Wilson and Mary Beth Lagerborg, *Once-a-Month Cooking* describes "A Time-Saving, Budget-Stretching Plan To Prepare Delicious Meals," sometimes called marathon cooking. Detailed menu plans and shopping lists tell you all you need to know for shopping and meal preparation, two to four weeks at a time. Send a donation of $9.00 (postage and handling included) to Focus on the Family, Colorado Springs, CO 80995.

Ortho Problem Solver

This huge volume contains a listing of every university (county) extension service in the U.S., plus much, much more. You can find *Ortho Problem Solver* at many home and garden centers.

Square Foot Gardening

Mel Bartholomew's book shows you how to make the most of your garden space. Published by Rodale Press, it's available through local libraries, home and garden centers and bookstores.

Thrifty Business: 111 Money Saving Tips

Rhonda Barfield's *classic* booklet, 32 pages, tells you how to save on groceries, supplies, clothes, some major household purchases, and recreation. $4.00 includes postage and handling, plus a guarantee that you'll save at least $40 or your money back. Send a check or money order to TB/B, P.O. Box 665, St. Charles, MO 63302-0665.

The $30 a Week Grocery Budget, Volume I
The $30 a Week Grocery Budget, Volume II

Donna McKenna's first volume sells for $5.00, the second, slightly-shorter volume for $4.50, postage and handling included. The first contains detailed information on how Donna feeds a family of six for $30 a week, the second, more general advice on saving money. Both books are worth the price if only for the low-cost recipes. Write to Donna at RR1 Box 189, Casco, ME 04015.

The Tightwad Gazette

The first two years of this popular newsletter by Amy Dacyzyn are now in book form, published by Villard Books, an imprint of Random House, Inc. Check your local library or bookstore.

The Use-It-Up Cookbook

Lois Carlson Willand has written 190 pages, a "Guide for Minimizing Food Waste," that shows how to creatively recycle every food imaginable. Send $9.75 (tax and postage included) to Practical Cookbooks, 145 Malcolm Avenue S.E., Minneapolis, MN 55414.

Food Stores
Aldi Inc.

As of this writing, there are 342 stores in 10 states. Call the divisional headquarters nearest you to find the closest store:

Illinois, Batavia: (708) 879-8100
Indiana, Greenwood: ((317) 885-0808
Indiana, Valparaiso: (219) 464-2500
Iowa, Burlington: (319) 753-6213
Kansas, Olathe: (913) 764-8822
Missouri, O'Fallon: (314) 278-4700
Ohio, Hinckley: (216) 273-7351

Save-A-Lot Food Stores

This food chain is similar to Aldi, but carries a larger selection of foods and is located in some areas where Aldi is not. Currently there are 380 stores in 21 states, most of them east of the Mississippi. For more information, call the national headquarters at 1-800-346-3808.

Newsletters
The Banker's Secret Bulletin

A quarterly newsletter dedicated to helping readers save money on their debts, like credit card bills and mortgages, subscriptions cost $19.95. Or send $1.00 for a bulletin sample to Good Advice Press, Box 78, Dept. EW, Elizaville, NY 12523.

Cheapskate Monthly

For a free newsletter sample, send a first-class stamp to Mary Hunt, P.O. Box 2135, Dept. EW, Paramount, CA 90723. Information about Mary Ann Maring, coupon queen, is found in issue #11, which costs $1.50. To subscribe, send $12.95 for 12 issues.

The Frugal Times

Adrianne Ferree recently sold her newsletter to *The Penny Pincher* (see two paragraphs below), but back issues are still available. Information about both Adrianne's system of monthly meal preparation and warehouse buying are found in issue #2; send an SASE to Jackie Iglehart (below) to find out how to purchase this and other back issues.

Living Cheap News

Larry Roth's newsletter contains general information on ways to save money. Send $1.00 and a self-addressed, stamped envelope for a sample copy, or $12 for a one year (10 issue) subscription, to Box 700058, Dept. EW, San Jose, CA 95170.

The Penny Pincher

Send a first-class stamp for a free newsletter sample and an index of already-published articles. Back issues sell for $2.00 each (through 12/92). Issue #5 explains breadmakers, including an ordering address and discount available to readers. Issue #7 has a recipe for homemade seltzer that costs only eight cents per liter. An annual subscription of 12 issues costs $12.00. Write to Jackie Iglehart, PO Box 809, Dept. EW, Kings Park, NY 11754.

Refund Express

If you're interested in large-scale couponing and refunding, send $3.00 for a sample issue of *Refund Express* to Sandy Ennis, P.O. Box 10, Allen Park, MI 48101.

Refunding Makes Cents! (RMC)

While you're at it, write to *RMC* for a slightly different approach to couponing and refunding. Send $2.95 for a sample issue to Michele Easter, Box R, Farmington, UT 84025.

Skinflint News

Enclose an extra stamped, self-addressed envelope in your envelope, and receive a free newsletter sample. Or send $9.95 for an annual (12 issue) subscription to Ron and Melodie Moore, 1460 Noell Boulevard, Dept. EW, Palm Harbor, FL 34683-5639.

Organizations and More
American Community Gardening Association

To learn more about opportunities for shared urban gardening, write to ACGA at 325 Walnut Street, Philadelphia, PA 19106.

International Reciprocal Trade Association

IRTA will help you locate bartering exchanges in your area. Send a self-addressed, stamped envelope to International Reciprocal Trade Association, 9513 Beach Mill Road, Great Falls, VA 22066 for more information.

La Leche League

For information on breastfeeding, answers to breastfeeding questions, a free catalog and/or the location of a nearby chapter, call 1-800-LALECHE.

Library System (Interlibrary Loans)

If you cannot find a book at the local library, request an interlibrary loan. Staff members will first try to locate a copy of the book in libraries nearby, then within your county or state. They will even make a nationwide search if necessary. Usually there is no cost to you.

National Cancer Institute

To receive free brochures on nutrition, including the "5 a Day for Better Health" plan, call 1-800-4-CANCER.

National Center for Nutrition and Dietetics of The American Dietetic Association

The Consumer Nutrition Hot Line, 1-800-366-1655, is a 24 hour service where consumers listen to recorded messages on current nutrition topics (both Spanish and English messages are available). From 9 to 4 CST you can also speak in person with a registered dietician or be referred to a registered dietician in your area. When you call, ask about ordering a copy of *The New Lean Toward Health*.

National Cooperative Business Association

For a free information packet on cooperatives and up-to-date information on cooperatives in your area, write to NCBA at 1401 New York Avenue, N.W., Suite 1100, Washington, DC 20005-2160.

National Cooperative Exchange

To learn more about bartering exchanges, write to the current president of the National Association of Trade Exchanges, Mark Tracy, at American Commerce Exchange, 10558 Riverside Drive, Toluca Lake, CA 91602.

National Council of State Garden Clubs

Write to the national headquarters at 4401 Magnolia Avenue, St. Louis, Missouri 63110-3492, or call (314) 776-7574 for information on the club nearest you in your state.

SHARE (Self Help & Resource Exchange)

Headquartered in San Diego, California, SHARE is currently located in18 states, some of them serving a several-states area: Arizona, California, Colorado, Florida, Georgia, Illinois, Kansas, Maryland, Massachusetts, Michigan, Minnesota, New York, New Jersey, North Carolina, Ohio, Pennsylvania, Virginia and Wisconsin. New chapters are being added, so call or write SHARE to locate the one nearest you. Call (619) 525-2200 or write SHARE, 6950 Friars Street, San Diego, CA 92108.

U.S. Department of Agriculture (USDA)

Write to Human Nutrition Information Service, Public Information Office, 364 Federal Building, 6506 Belcrest Road, Hyattsville, MD 20782, or call 301-436-8617 for free information on a variety of nutritional subjects.

U.S. Cooperative Food Warehouses

The National Cooperative Business Association currently lists the following contacts as regional sources for co-op buying. If you find an address or phone number is no longer correct, please contact the NCBA for up-to-date information.

Northeastern States
Hudson Valley Federation
P.O. Box 367
Clintondale, NY 12515
914/883-6848

Northeast Cooperatives, Inc.
P.O. Box 8188, Quinn Road
Brattleboro, VT 05304
802/257-5856

Southeastern States
Orange Blossom Warehouse
1601 N.W. 55th Place
Gainesville, FL 32606
904/372-7061

Midwestern States
Blooming Prairie Warehouse, Inc.
2340 Heinz Road
Iowa City, IA 52240
319/337-6448

Federation of Ohio River
Cooperatives
320-E Outerbelt, Suite E
Columbus, OH 43213
614/861-2446

North Farm Co-op Warehouse
204 Regas Road
Madison, WI 53714
608/241-2667

Ozark Co-op Warehouse
Box 1528
Fayetteville, AR 72702
501/521-4920

Western States
Associated Cooperatives, Inc.
12250 San Pablo Avenue, #155
Richmond, CA 94805-2453
415/232-1111

Tucson Cooperative Warehouse
350 S. Toole
Tucson, AZ 85701
602/884-9951

INDEX

Note: Some printed materials, grocery stores, newsletters, organizations and food warehouses not listed in this index can be found in Resources, pages 135-142.

Did you borrow this book? Or would you like to share your copy with a friend?

Please enclose $9.95 + $2.50 postage & handling to
Lilac Publishing, P.O. Box 665, St. Charles, MO 63302-0665.

Name

Address

City   State   Zip

Phone

Your satisfaction is guaranteed!
Discounts available for orders
of 10 or more books.

Number of Books Ordered	
Subtotal for Books	
Postage $2.50 for first book 50¢ each additional book	
MO res. add 7.22%	
Grand Total	

RECIPE INDEX